HATHA YOGA PRADIPIKA

Light on Hatha Yoga

HATHA YOGA PRADIPIKA

Light on Hatha Yoga

Commentary by

YOGI HARI

NADA PRODUCTIONS, INC.

For information address: NADA PRODUCTIONS INC., 12750 SW 33ST.,
Miramar, FL 33027, Tel. (954) 843-0319, 1-800-964-2553.

www.yogihari.com
www.yoga-sampoorna.org
shriyogihari@aol.com
ISBN: 1-57777-052-8
First edition 5,000 copies
Library of Congress Control Number 2001012345

DEDICATION

*This book is dedicated to all my Gurus from ancient time
to my present incarnation*

ACKNOWLEDGEMENTS

My prayers, blessings and deep appreciation to the following individuals whose unselfish contributions of expertise and resources made this project possible.

Isabel Riesco for the design and layout of the book and cover.

Beth Rosen (Bhagavati) for her tireless editing and proofreading of the text.

Elizabeth Chene for her unwavering support and kind words in the foreword.

Sybille and Gopala for typing.

Vinu Patel of Zimbabwe for donating the funds for this publication without any hesitation or conditions.

FOREWORD

There are many who have crossed Sri Yogi Hari's path. They probably experienced his enchanting voice, enlivening kirtan, peaceful charm, poise, incredible flexibility and beautiful Yoga postures. Most of them, however, consumed and distracted again with worldly matters such as occupation and material pursuits, have missed something very sacred.

Those who were fortunate to go beyond these external expressions and study under his tutelage were graced with the essence of a loving Sage and a venerable Rishi. Having studied with him for many years, I can attest to his dedication and selfless service to uplift humanity. Notwithstanding our mistakes and misunderstandings, Sri Yogi Hari, in his infinite compassion and wisdom, is always willing to lend a helping hand and gently guide us back on the right track toward Self-Realization. He is not only a Master experienced in Sadhana, but he lives his life in accordance with the Scriptures and true Yogic values, modeling to us the role of a divine and devoted husband, father and Guru. His main concern over the past 30 years has been to share the wealth of the science of Yoga with his students and serious aspirants.

Everything Sri Yogi Hari has produced thus far has been done in the spirit of service. With the help of today's technology, he has used his divine gifts and all his resources to make readily available the traditional tools of Yoga in all their purity. Without his dedication, genuine enthusiasm and interest in the uplifting of humanity, the ancient secrets of Yoga and the wealth of treasures he has produced would have remained lost, hidden or otherwise forgotten. The variety of CD's,

DVD's, videos and books on Nada Yoga and Hatha Yoga produced through Nada Productions Inc. are invaluable resources for those who sincerely strive to regain their physical and mental balance, improve their concentration, rid themselves of negative emotions, enhance their understanding of yogic values and live a meaningful and fulfilling life.

Steadfast in his convictions, Sri Yogi Hari never compromises what he knows from the depth of his heart and from his own experience to be absolute truth. Notwithstanding the current trends to conjure up flashy, new and improved spiritual paths and techniques that pollute even the world of Yoga today, Sri Yogi Hari teaches Yoga in its pure form as passed down from Guru to disciple from ancient times. Frozen knowledge and superstitious beliefs have no hold on him because he truly lives in the present moment.

This commentary on *Hatha Yoga Pradipika* is the latest evidence of his dedication to service and truth. Here, he provides an easily readable and usable version of this sacred Scripture, which is designed to bring Yoga back into its proper perspective so that aspirants can access this divine gift for their highest spiritual evolution. This commentary is predicated on his profound experience and sound common sense. Holding firmly to absolute truth and refusing to be swayed by misinterpretations that have been perpetuated over time, Sri Yogi Hari takes a bold step with this truly divine project. This commentary puts aspirants back on track. From time to time, Masters come to teach humanity and re-light the path so that people can find their way back home. This commentary is the lighthouse that directs the ships lost at sea back to land. Have the courage to turn away from the half and incomplete truths that inundate the commercial field of Hatha Yoga today and read this incredibly sacred book.

Foreword

I have been practicing Yoga for 30 years and teaching for 23 years. For the past 8 years, I have had the divine privilege to follow Sri Yogi Hari as his disciple. I can say from the depth of my soul that this book is a precious gift, living proof of the Guru's constant support and love to enable us to continue to progress in the right direction. But to truly appreciate the value of this divine commentary, we must, however, remember that the Scriptures and teachings of a Master are not mere food for thought. They are meant to be savored, digested and assimilated. Just as a flower reveals its fragrance as you step closer and closer to it, the same is true with the techniques divulged in this book. When they are approached step-by-step, assimilated, absorbed and put into practice, over time you will discover a new universal dimension opening as they reveal themselves in all their richness.

Contrary to an ordinary book that you may read once, place on the bookshelf and forget about, this book is a daily resource, one that you can read over and over. It is designed to nourish the soul and provide many avenues for reflection and meditation, faithfully guiding us beyond our limitations until we reach the ultimate goal of liberation, to experience absolute Truth. May we all reach this goal with God's and Guru's blessings.

Elizabeth Chene

CONTENTS

WHY THIS BOOK?

Throughout the ages, enlightened Masters have provided perfect teachings that serve as a road map to take spiritual aspirants to the goal of enlightenment. Even though Masters expound absolute truth, students can only grasp knowledge according to their level of awareness. As long as the Master is present, he can guide aspirants in the right direction. While some may elevate their consciousness, only a few will reach the ultimate goal of enlightenment and liberation. That is why, as time goes by, teachings degenerate. Compromises are made and people adjust the teachings to suit their conveniences.

This is what happened to the teachings of Buddha, Jesus, Shankaracharya and other great Masters. The same thing happened with respect to the knowledge of Hatha Yoga. Even though it was Lord Shiva himself who bestowed the science of Hatha Yoga with the sole purpose of elevating people to the state of perfection, as time marched on, a great deal of confusion arose as to the real truth about the teachings. That is why the great Master, Yogi Swatmarama decided to set humanity and aspirants back on the right track through a systematic outline of the practice called "*Hatha Yoga Pradipika*," which means "light on Hatha Yoga."

As it is the nature and fate of teachings, today we find ourselves in the same condition as the one that prompted Yogi Swatmarama to throw some light on this science. We have once again reached a state of confusion about what Hatha Yoga really is, resulting in conflicting interpretations of the Scriptures on the practice as outlined by Yogi Swatmarama.

In spite of the extensive dissemination of information on Hatha Yoga in terms of books and other mediums of communication, the people who commented on *Hatha Yoga Pradipika* are, for the most part, not experienced enough in the actual practice of Hatha Yoga. They are Sanskrit scholars who merely interpret the words and prescribe meanings that make sense to them but which do not necessarily convey the truth about the science. Some may dabble in Hatha Yoga but they do not immerse themselves in the actual practice. It takes someone with thorough understanding and extensive experience of the subject to make it comprehensible to people in light of present day expression.

Hatha Yoga is a science that is meant to take the aspirant to the state of perfection. The truth that Swatmarama outlined in his day and age is the same today. That truth is stipulated in the very beginning of the *Hatha Yoga Pradipika*, which explains the purpose of Hatha Yoga. The very first Sloka states that it was Adinath or Shiva, the first God and Guru, who gave the knowledge as a step-by-step process for one to reach the highest state of realization, the highest state of union, the highest state of Yoga, which is called Raja Yoga. On the basis of this Sloka, almost all the commentators that I have examined make the preliminary mistake of concluding that Hatha Yoga is nothing more than a preparation for the practice of Raja Yoga. The misunderstanding stems from the use of the words "Raja Yoga." But to dispel any confusion on this matter, in the fourth chapter, verses 3 and 4, it is very clearly stated that, "Raja Yoga, Samadhi, Unmani, Manonmani, Amaratwa, Laya, Sahaja, Tattva, Shunyashunya, Parampadam, Amanaskam, Adwaitam, Niralamba, Niranjana, Jivanmukti and Turiya are all synonymous terms." Thus, in this context, the term "Raja Yoga" is clearly used to mean a state of transcendence or perfection rather than a system of practice.

There is, of course, a lot of preparation to be done in order to reach a point in life when one is able to practice Yoga as outlined in the *Hatha Yoga Pradipika*. As presented there, it is meant for people with certain qualifications, who have fulfilled their obligations to family and society, and who are ready to retire from the world. But this does not preclude others from practicing Hatha Yoga. In the meantime, people can practice certain disciplines to help them maintain good health. In Hatha Yoga classes, they can experience exercise, breathing and relaxation, which if done properly, will alleviate the stress that day-to-day life imposes on them. When incorporated with proper diet and positive thinking, such disciplines will lead to good health and peace of mind, which may inspire some to pursue other yogic disciplines and further elevate their consciousness.

It is important to keep in mind that the science of liberation is not confined solely to good physical and mental health, though these are necessary prerequisities. These teachings are specifically meant for those who have fulfilled their obligations and duties in society; who have attained enough economic freedom; whose minds are fully withdrawn from the external world; and who can retire in an Ashram to live a life of a Yogi in seclusion. At that stage, their desire is to fully focus on their Sadhana (spiritual practice) as instructed by a Guru who has proper understanding of the science as outlined in the *Hatha Yoga Pradipika*.

A person who is worthy or capable of such a discipline is someone who has lived a dharmic life (a life based on moral and ethical discipline) and does not have to struggle with the ethical and moral laws known as Yamas and Niyamas. When the *Hatha Yoga Pradipika* declares that Asana (Yoga posture) is the first practice, it is assuming that the person is already established in Yamas and Niyamas, which are actually the starting point and foundation for all spiritual disciplines.

To draw an analogy, if you want to learn how to sing, the first thing you have to practice is the notes of the musical scale. It is not necessary to mention that you must have a voice or vocal cords to sing because it is taken for granted. Similarly, for one to reach the stage where one practices Hatha Yoga for enlightenment, the first discipline one has to practice is Asana. This implies that you have already incorporated values of straightforwardness, truthfulness, honesty, purity, love, compassion, generosity, forgiveness, tolerance, etc. in your life. Only a person with these qualities will have higher aspirations and a desire to practice discipline for Self-Realization and liberation. If you have not lived a dharmic, straightforward, truthful, honest, loving and kind life as outlined in the Scriptures, you will not have the aspiration to practice Yoga for enlightenment.

The mere fact that you have fulfilled your obligations means that you probably will have gone through the normal stages of life such as studentship, marriage, and professional career. In this context, not only will you have acquired secular knowledge, but you will also have had spiritual instructions and guidance from a Guru throughout your life, practicing the Yoga of Integration with a passion for Hatha Yoga. Because you have been living your life this way, by the time you retire, you are also blessed with radiant health, physically and mentally. You have not traded your health for wealth, thereby obviating the need to undergo physical and psychological therapy. Most people's involvement in Yoga is for rehabilitation from the abuse they suffered from living a life of indulgence and lack of awareness of the higher goal and purpose of life. But having gone through these stages of life with proper understanding and awareness of the true goal and purpose of life, one will experience a burning desire for liberation.

By the time you retire (the Vanaprastha stage), your mind is free from worldly matters and involvement. You will have attained economic independence or be able to rely on well wishers, family or disciples to provide for you so that you can live as a recluse without having to think about where you will get your food.

Having understood the kind of discipline that is recommended in the *Hatha Yoga Pradipika*, you will find that all your time will be spent in Sadhana. And in a society like ours, it is not practical to beg for food as it used to be, and to some extent still is, the tradition of spiritual people in India.

Of course, in every society and religion, there are people who have embraced monastic life without going through the natural stages of life first. These are people with strong monastic Samskaras from previous incarnations in which they practiced Sadhana and developed strong dispassion for the world. They do not feel the urge to go through the stages of having a family and a career, and can, as soon as they finish school, retire into an ashram and continue their Sadhana to reach the goal of enlightenment.

In this context, there is also a practical reason why the *Hatha Yoga Pradipika* has to be retold in present day understanding. It would not be practical to squat on any place in just any country you like and build a hermitage using cow dung according to Yogi Swatmarama's instructions. The owners of the property and the zoning, building and health officials would pound down your door. You would not have the solitude and peace of mind necessary for practicing Sadhana.

Because of the confusion about Yoga in this age, especially about Hatha Yoga, I have decided to shed some clear light on the *Hatha Yoga Pradipika*. Considering the misunderstandings about the purpose of Yoga and the misintepretation of the teachings, I saw the need for an up to date interpretation of this very sacred and important Scripture for those who desire liberation.

It must be understood from the very beginning that Hatha Yoga is a complete and step-by-step system to reach perfection. It is a scientific and systematic approach of refinement and purification on all levels: physical, pranic, emotional, mental and intellectual, resulting in complete identification with the Higher Self.

However, one can practice aspects of Hatha Yoga, such as Asanas, Pranayama and proper diet, as a preparation for Raja Yoga, Karma Yoga, Bhakti Yoga or any other kind of Yoga since you need proper health to do Sadhana. Hatha Yoga can be approached just for that purpose: to have a foundation for the practice of another discipline. But since this comes from a limited vantage point, one should not mistakenly limit Hatha Yoga's usefulness to only those certain components of Hatha Yoga. In actuality, Hatha Yoga is a full, complete system that is designed to take you to the goal of liberation.

Taking the Slokas literally, however, can lead to great superstition, such as viewing the practice of Hatha Yoga as a cure for all diseases. People consult a Yoga teacher as if they are consulting a doctor for a prescription, looking for a specific Asana to cure diabetes, high blood pressure, asthma, etc. Most people usually do not understood that the path of Yoga is a way of life to prepare the instrument for the higher awakening of consciousness and to reach the state of perfection. It is a systematic approach to realize your Divinity, your Self, or in other words, to know the answer to the question, "Who am I?"

It is from this perspective that I will expound on this sacred Scripture. The translation of the Slokas are, for the most part, clear and straight forward. I will therefore group Slokas together sometimes when commenting, particularly when they are related to one overall concept or practice. The whole outline as presented here sets forth a complete system of practice that is in keeping with the philosophy of Sampoorna Yoga, which is a holistic approach that works on every aspect of the personality and is in harmony with the teachings of Master Sivananda. I will explain the necessity and benefits of Asanas, right attitude, proper diet, Kriyas, Pranayama, Kumbhakas, Mudras and Bandhas, the breaking of knots to release the Kundalini Shakti, the experience of the Anahata sound and finally, the reaching of liberation or Raja Yoga through Samadhi. With this process in mind, the study of the *Hatha Yoga Pradipika* will provide you with an entirely new understanding of the practice of Hatha Yoga.

Chapter One

A S A N A S

1

SALUTATIONS TO THE FIRST GOD AND GURU SRI ADINATH WHO GAVE THE KNOWLEDGE OF HATHA YOGA AS A STEP-BY-STEP PROCESS TO REACH THE HIGHEST STATE OF PERFECTION, RAJA YOGA.

The first God and Guru is Shiva. Shiva is referred to as Adinath, which means the first Lord, and it is he who imparted this knowledge of Hatha Yoga to humanity. This knowledge was given by God himself as a stairway to reach the highest state of evolution, the highest state of realization, the highest state of Yoga, the experience of your Divine Self, referred to as Raja Yoga.

Raja Yoga here is not referred to as a system but rather as a state that one reaches through the systematic step-by-step practice, which is called Hatha Yoga. In fact, in chapter 4, verses 3 and 4, it is very clearly stated that, "Raja Yoga, Samadhi, Unmani, Manonmani, Amaratwa, Laya, Sahaja, Tattva, Shunyashunya, Parampadam, Amanaskam, Adwaitam, Niralamba, Niranjana, Jivanmukti and Turiya are all synonymous terms," which implies that the term Raja Yoga, as used here, is a state of perfection.

Now let us take a moment and think rationally and logically about this step-by-step practice, called Hatha Yoga, which will lead to Raja Yoga, or in other words, a state of perfection. If God is providing and outlining a system, what kind of system is that going to be? It is going to be perfect! It will not need anything else to complement it. He will not teach you something that is only partial. It will be "Sampoorna," a full and complete system to take you to the highest stage of Yoga, or in other words, the experience of your Divine Self.

Hatha Yoga is not given merely as a means for one to start the practice of another systematic Yogic discipline known as Raja Yoga. Hatha Yoga is a complete perfect system unto itself. This is where all the commentators that I have examined make their first mistake in interpreting the *Hatha Yoga Pradipika*. They misconstrue the meaning of Raja Yoga in the very beginning and therefore incorrectly conclude that Hatha Yoga is only a preparation for the practice of Raja Yoga. Because of this initial blunder, they become confused and cannot reconcile it in the rest of their exposition, which unfortunately misleads the reader and spiritual aspirants.

What is Yoga? It is the experience of the Oneness, that thou art that, just as a wave is one with the ocean and never separate from it. That state of Yoga can only be reached when the mind becomes completely purified and freed from all defects. In that state, the limitations of body, mind, intellect and relative world awareness are transcended, and one experiences their Divine Self.

This system called Hatha Yoga is a deliberate step-by-step path to take you to the highest state of evolution or experience. This is why Hatha Yoga is so effective. If it is practiced properly with right guidance and right understanding, you will discover that you will ascend gradually from one level to another. When people do not understand that it is a perfect system to reach a state of perfection, they reduce the practice of Hatha Yoga to mere physical exercises and postures. That is the biggest blunder of most people practicing Hatha Yoga today. And that is where it will remain unless someone sheds light on the matter to regain what was lost in translation and commentary. Hatha Yoga does not need anything else to complement or supplement it. It is a perfect system in itself that can take you to the state of enlightenment and liberation.

2
YOGI SWATMARAMA, HAVING INVOKED THE BLESSINGS OF THE GURU, GAVE THE KNOWLEDGE OF HATHA YOGA FOR THE ATTAINMENT OF PERFECTION.

A truly cultured person always begins a project by first invoking the blessings of God and Guru for inspiration and success. Yogi Swatmarama, being an enlightened Master, first pays due respect and homage to Shiva, the source of this knowledge, and to his Guru through whom this knowledge flowed.

This inspiration is flowing from the Guru, who is the Lord, because he is in contact with the Cosmic Mind. If there is no reverence and devotion for the Guru, then you will remain with a mind that is veiled and whatever you express will be from your ego. But if you have true reverence and devotion for the Guru who you behold as God himself, who came in this human form to teach you and to shed the light of knowledge in order to dispel the darkness of ignorance, then you will create the necessary condition in your mind to connect with the Cosmic Mind.

This is why, before starting any project of learning and teaching, there is so much emphasis placed on prostration and reverence for the Guru. If you see the Guru as a man sitting before you, then that is what he will be. In that case, you will get instructions and information from a person. But if you see that Guru as God who is there to remove your ignorance, then you will have the kind of surrender, faith and devotion, where transformation will take place from every single word that flows through him.

Spiritual knowledge and enlightenment is not possible without a Guru. All the Scriptures and enlightened Masters confirm this. Only ignorant people and certain tabloid magazines proclaim otherwise. Of course, if your aim and goal is only six pack abs and buns of steel, you do not need a Guru.

Twice already, Yogi Swatmarama declares that the purpose of Hatha Yoga is to lead you to the highest state of perfection.

3
BECAUSE OF CONFUSION AND MISUNDERSTANDING OF HATHA YOGA, COMPASSIONATE YOGI SWATMARAMA DECIDED TO THROW LIGHT ON THIS SUBJECT.

Unfortunately, confusion and misunderstanding is the human condition. No matter how lofty and perfect the teaching of the Master, the moment he is removed, everyone starts to interpret according to their own condition and state of consciousness. Therefore, it degenerates more and more and becomes confusing. Even today, disciples coming from the same Master are quarreling, bickering and fighting about who is teaching the right tutelage of the Master. This occurred in ancient times, it happens today, and it will continue to happen in the future. Throughout history, you find the same misconceptions, misunderstandings and misinterpretations. Therefore, someone will appear from time to time who has gone through the process and experienced the knowledge to put the record straight, to remove the misconceptions and to relight the path.

The truth is not invented, it is just retold and restated. In different times, circumstances and ages, it is restated in different ways to suit people's understanding, which means in whatever terms they can comprehend. If you are speaking to a scientist, you will use scientific terms. You may talk about atoms, molecules, protons, neutrons and electrons. If you are speaking to a farmer, you will speak in terms of plowing the soil and sowing seeds. But it is the same truth that you are expressing. Now you can express the same truth that conveys the same meaning or you can have a misunderstanding and convey something quite opposite or contrary to what it should be.

In every age, Masters come to retell the truth, to remove the misconceptions and misunderstandings. The absolute truth is the same. It always has been, is, and will continue to be the same. We find ourselves in the same plight today concerning Hatha Yoga, which is why this project is extremely necessary and important.

4

MATSYENDRANATH, GORAKHNATH AND OTHERS HAD A THOROUGH KNOWLEDGE OF HATHA YOGA AND THROUGH THEIR GRACE, YOGI SWATMARAMA LEARNED IT.

We know from the Puranas that Matsyendranath was the first recipient of this knowledge. When Shiva and Parvati were in their mountain resort in Mount Kailas, Parvati, because of her compassionate nature as the mother who is always looking after the interest of her offspring, saw the children in this creation suffering and asked, "Father, isn't there something we can do to ease the suffering of our children, of humanity?" He answered, "Yes! Sit and listen."

Shiva closed his eyes, and from the state of intuition, the perfect knowledge of Hatha Yoga flowed. When he opened his eyes, he saw Parvati sleeping and thought, "What a waste!" But then he looked in the lake and saw a fish very attentive, drinking in all the knowledge. He smiled, blessed the fish and the fish became Matsyendranath. So Matsyendranath became the first recipient of this knowledge and he gave the knowledge to Gorakhnath and others.

The mystical significance of this story is important. Shiva is pure consciousness, which is "Sat-Chit-Ananda," absolute existence, knowledge and bliss. Parvati represents Prakriti, the universal Divine Mother or Nature. One who identifies with body, mind and intellect in the waking, dreaming and deep sleep state of consciousness is, in fact, existing in a sleeping state. However, when the individual aspires for self knowledge that will free him from this relative and dualistic state of existence, which is synonymous with suffering and bondage, he develops that devotion and one pointed concentration. This is what the fish represents. It never blinks or sleeps. This penetrating ability will enable him to reach a state of intuition in which absolute knowledge from the cosmic mind is revealed. In other words, he is blessed by Shiva and is transformed from the lower consciousness to that of a Divine being, Matsyendranath.

LINEAGE

5-9

SHIVA, MATSYENDRA, SHABARA, ANANDABHAIRAVA, CHAURANGI, MINA, GORAKSHA, VIRUPAKSHA, BILESHAYA, MANTHANA, BHAIRAVA, SIDDHI, BUDDHA, KANTHADI, KORANTAKA, SURANANDA, SIDDHIPADA, CHARAP- ATI, KANERI, PUJYAPADA, NITYANATH, NIRANJAN, KAPALI, BINDUNATH, KAKACHANDISHWARA, ALLAMA, PRABHUDEVA, GHODACHOLI, TINTINI, BHANUKI, NARADEVA, KHANDA, KAPALIKA AND OTHERS ARE PERFECT- ED MASTERS WHO, HAVING CONQUERED DEATH THROUGH THE PRAC- TICE OF HATHA YOGA, ROAM THE UNIVERSE.

This is the line of Gurus, Siddhas or Enlightened Masters, through whom the perfect knowledge of Yoga flowed until it reached Yogi Swatmarama. It is through the practice of Hatha Yoga that they were able to obtain immortality and can now roam the universe. Can you name anyone who was able to conquer death by simply doing Asana practice? How would you reach immortality by doing Asanas? These Slokas do not, in any way, suggest that one must first practice Hatha Yoga as if it were merely the practice of Asanas and then move onto another discipline, namely Raja Yoga, in order to reach immortality. It simply states that the means to immortality is through Hatha Yoga, indicating a complete system to realize your Oneness with the Supreme Consciousness.

Once you reach that highest state of perfection or identify completely with your Divine Immortal Self, you transcend death. The statement, "They roam about the universe," means that they are omnipresent. You will find that the kind of energy you tap into depends on your state of consciousness. If you reach the stage where you exhaust the knowledge of ordinary teachers, you can tune into the cosmic mind and access inspiration and knowledge from the Masters as they roam about the universe helping people. Just as Einstein is not going to teach a kindergarten child mathematics, these Masters are not simply going to teach people how to lift their legs! You do not need Yogi Swatmarama for that.

10 •
JUST AS A HOUSE PROTECTS ONE FROM THE SCORCHING HEAT OF THE SUN, HATHA YOGA PROTECTS ONE FROM THE THREE TAPAS AND FOR THOSE WHO ARE INTENSE IN THEIR PRACTICE, HATHA YOGA ACTS LIKE A TORTOISE SUPPORTING THE WORLD.

The Tapas or suffering referred to here is of three kinds: Adibhautika, which is suffering caused by other beings, Adhidevika, which is suffering caused by nature, and Adhyatmika, which is suffering caused by oneself.

Every being in this world experiences pain that is caused by other beings such as deminic people, animals, insects, reptiles, viruses, bacteria, etc. Whether you are outside or inside, insects are constantly creating all kinds of disease and sickness. Not only are your pets shedding all kind of diseases but you are ingesting them. Harmful bacteria and viruses exist everywhere ready to unleash suffering and pain. This is known as Adibhautika or suffering caused by other beings.

Adhidevika means suffering caused by nature, referred to by the ancients as Devatas. Floods, hurricanes, tornados, earthquakes, extreme heat and extreme cold are examples of Devatas. People in the north often suffer from extreme cold and some people even die from it. You can find this kind of suffering everywhere. I never met anybody who said that he enjoyed the bitter cold or scorching heat. Often when there is inclement weather, you have to protect yourself from it.

Next there is Adhyatmika, suffering that is created by yourself through ignorance, lack of knowledge, wrong conditioning, wrong identification and not knowing the true goal and purpose of life. Thus, you unwittingly and continuously abuse the gift of the body, the gift that God has given you. You abuse your emotions, your senses and your mind. Often, you employ your intellect for the wrong purpose, such as becoming more immersed in lust, hatred and jealousy. Therefore, you constantly suffer.

The science of Hatha Yoga can help you to live a life of balance amidst all these trials and hardships. It bestows knowledge and provides you with a better way of living that brings you into harmony with yourself, others, the environment and the universe so that you are no longer vulnerable to pain and suffering.

For instance, you can improve your health, resistance and immune system through the discipline of Hatha Yoga. It helps to strengthen the mind and will so that you are no longer victimized by the flu and the myriad of physical discomforts, emotional swings, mental turmoil, imbalances and other medical problems that people experience. By living in harmony with nature, you are able to experience a state of ease and balance.

People who are intense in their practice and experiencing all kinds of phenomena, like sudden surges of energy without knowing how to channel it, may use it for the wrong purpose which will create more problems. For those people, this science acts like a tortoise, or in other words, a support.

This analogy is given in the Puranas where the Demons and the Devas were engaged in the project of churning the ocean of milk to obtain the nectar of immortality. The Gods were on one side and the Demons on the other side as they used Mount Meeru as the churning rod and the eternal serpent Vasuki as the churning rope. As they churned, the mountain descended deep into the ocean. If they continued churning as such, they risked devastating the entire universe. Therefore Vishnu came as a tortoise, known as "Kurmavatar," where he became the support on which the mountain rested, enabling them to continue churning and be successful.

This illustrates that if God and Guru are not your support, then your practice can lead to devastation. When Kundalini Shakti begins to awaken and you start to experience the effects of your practice, you would be lost, not knowing what to do, because you are delving into realms of mind, emotions and consciousness itself, unleashing energy of which you have no understanding.

11
A YOGI WHO DESIRES SUCCESS IN HATHA YOGA SHOULD KEEP HIS PRACTICE A SECRET. IF REVEALED, IT LOSES ITS EFFECTIVENESS.

You should continuously strive to refine yourself and your personality and to reduce the ego. The tendency of most people is to tread the spiritual path for a short while and then the moment they experience a little bit of knowledge and understanding, they want to show off to their friends. They seek glorification, acceptance and praise, looking for feedback about how much they have changed. This is the natural tendency of people. But in the process of doing that, a person's ego can easily become his biggest obstacle. Thus, some get stuck in certain areas and they do not continue to progress. Maintaining one's practice as a secret helps to curb the natural tendency to want to show off to others. Let's face it: everybody wants to be a Guru, very few want to be a disciple and even fewer want to be disciplined.

If you desire to be wealthy, you have to save and continue to accumulate more wealth. If you spend and squander your money, you will never realize your goal of being wealthy. Similarly, if you want to be successful in the practice of Hatha Yoga, you have to spend your time in Sadhana and not waste your time in boastful demonstrations. It will not add to your progress. Instead, it will only serve to inflate your ego.

HERMITAGE- LOCATION

12
A YOGI SHOULD LIVE ALONE AND PRACTICE IN A HERMITAGE THAT IS SAFE FROM HAZARDS OF FALLEN ROCKS, FOREST FIRES AND FLOODS. THE COUNTRY, STATE OR TOWN SHOULD BE PROSPEROUS WITH RELIGIOUS TOLERANCE. THE CITIZENS SHOULD SUPPORT HERMITS AND MONKS THROUGH CHARITY AND ALMSGIVING.

Clearly, the practitioners who have reached this stage in their life have fulfilled all their social and family obligations. As students, they not only excelled in secular education but grew up with proper understanding as to the true goal and purpose of life. They have a Guru who taught them Yoga and Sadhana. They clearly understand the four treasures of life (Dharma, Artha, Kama and Moksha). Therefore in their Grihastha stage (family life), they apply this teaching, living a dharmic life and fulfilling all their family and social obligations while continuing their Sadhana of Hatha Yoga to maintain good health and balance in life. Those people who have fulfilled all their obligations and developed dispassion for the world can retire in a hermitage or Ashram to intensify their practice of Hatha Yoga under the guidance of their Guru and as outlined in the *Hatha Yoga Pradipika*.

On the other hand, there are young people who, by virtue of their state of evolution, know that they do not need to go through the normal stages of life like Grihastha, family life, etc., and they delight in Sadhana. They know that they are not victims or puppets of their emotions and senses. They really aspire and long for liberation and want to know the truth. They too can retire.

The people who have reached the stage of evolution where they have strength and steadiness of mind, dispassion for the world and longing for liberation, can retire and live alone. Living in your hermitage means that you live by yourself in seclusion to do your Sadhana. You will discover that living with others is always distracting. It does not matter if it is only one person. You will still have to adjust your life to suit them. You will be guided or conditioned by time and schedule, considering the other person each time you do something. You must ask yourself, "Am I disturbing them?" Even if the relationship is harmonious, there is still a subtle psychological impediment.

Living alone helps you to withdraw your mind completely and to focus your mind on your Sadhana. You also want to live where there are no "hazards," meaning where there is no danger of rocks or trees falling on you or insects or snakes biting you. Because when you are meditating or doing your Sadhana, if your mind is on disaster or potential disasters, then naturally your mind will be distracted from your practice. The objective is to remove agitation from the mind.

Today, especially in Westernized cultures, this Sloka can be construed to mean that you should live away from the noise, pollution and constant agitation of city life since it can be very distracting. It is a practical thing, not at all mysterious or mystical.

You will also want to live in a country where you will not be persecuted for your practice, or be perceived as a terrorist or a potential danger. There are countries where you cannot practice Yoga because they will incarcerate you. How can you practice in such a place? Your mind will be in a constant state of anxiety and fear.

Now, at this point in your life, you have ceased working in a job or business. Instead, you depend on alms. You are not going to waste your time with cooking or shopping in the market. To go shopping, you need money, to get money, you need to work, and so on. Then there will be no time for Sadhana as prescribed in this Scripture.

When you think about taking alms, there may appear to be a contradiction with the sattwic diet Yogi Swatmarama outlines later, because you must take whatever food is given to you. But what is implied here is that you should live where good alms can be easily attained, in a place where your practice is supported and alms giving is readily acceptable as part of the culture or tradition since it would not suffice for you to receive just any kind of alms. You certainly would not want to eat leftovers that someone would not even give to their pet dog. If you have fulfilled your duties properly, most likely people in your family will take care of you, or if you are a Guru, your disciples will support you with love and caring. You will make sure that you get the right food at the right time and you will not have to beg. Even now when people in India know that a Sadhu is doing Tapas, they bring him food so that he does not have to beg. If these details are not attended to, you will be wasting your life and time with small things.

HERMITAGE - DESCRIPTION

13

**THE DESCRIPTION OF THE HERMITAGE AS PRESCRIBED BY THE SID-
DHAS IS AS FOLLOWS: A SMALL DOOR FOR ENTRANCE AND NO WIN-
DOWS OR HOLES. IT SHOULD NOT BE TOO HIGH OR TOO LOW. IT MUST
BE SPOTLESSLY CLEAN, WIPED WITH COW MANURE AND FREE FROM
ANIMALS AND INSECTS. IT SHOULD HAVE A VERANDA, A WELL AND BE
SURROUNDED BY A WALL OR FENCE. THE APPEARANCE SHOULD BE
PLEASANT.**

Everything mentioned here has a practical purpose. These instructions were meant
for that specific time period and for poor countries lacking the affluence of the
West. In fact, this is how the majority of people in the world still live. They build
houses with tatched roof, mud floor and use cow dung and mud to construct the
walls. To prevent dust from accumulating, they use a mixture of cow dung with
clay and water and smear the floor with it, which seals all the dust. The cow dung
also acts as an insecticide, preventing infestation from insects and ants. It is not the
kind of cow dung that you have here in the West or other affluent countries where
the cow feed consists of artificial food with animal products. This makes the dung
toxic with a stench odor. In poor countries, the cows eat grass, which gives the cow
manure a pleasant odor. But do not take this Sloka literally. You do not need to
import cow dung from India into your room to feel that you are practicing authen-
tic Yoga.

With respect to more affluent countries, this can be interpreted to mean that you
live in a nice convenient place, where you can be secluded in your home with nice
carpet on the floor and blinds on your windows. The reason why it is recommended that the hermitage have no windows or holes is to prevent your mind from
wandering to the constant distraction of the scenery outside. Otherwise you will

be glancing out the window, noticing the sun, thinking to yourself how nice the weather is and then wanting to go outside and enjoy it.

Your house must be free from animals and insects. Some people practice with their cat or dog, thinking that it is so nice that their pet is doing Yoga with them! But cats and dogs are not doing Yoga. They will only serve to distract you from your practice.

And of course you do not have to go outside and drink well water since you have nice running water! All the conveniences of modern day technology are at your fingertips. Thus, there should be no excuse for you not to do Sadhana.

Finally, the appearance of the hermitage should be pleasant. You do not want people to feel it is a spooky, haunted place where a strange person is involved in some questionable practice.

14
LIVING IN THIS HERMITAGE, THE YOGI BEING FREE OF ANXIETY SHOULD PRACTICE YOGA AS TAUGHT BY HIS GURU.

When you are in seclusion, with no distraction and the mind is indrawn, with no television playing in the background or people to distract you, you can practice your Sadhana as instructed by your Guru. It does not mean that the Guru must always be with you physically.

For example, my Guru taught me a plethora of music. I could spend the rest of my life perfecting it. Once I had the foundation and knew all the rules and disciplines, he did not have to stay with me continuously. Of course if I had questions, I could approach him. The Guru is available when you need clarification.

It is very important to practice as instructed by your Guru. Today, if you teach a little bit of Asana or Pranayama to people, they lack that faith and trust to do exactly as you instruct them. Instead, at the onset of their practice, they want to do their own thing with their own variation because they want to be a Guru. People like that do not get too far because they are lacking the necessary faith and trust in the Guru and the wisdom behind everything that he is teaching. If you understand the wisdom behind his teachings, you will have trust and faith to practice according to his instructions. You will become established in that practice and then later on, if things start to flow and you need to adapt for whatever purpose, condition or situation, then it will be okay to make modifications. In fact, if you continue for awhile as instructed by your Guru and lift your consciousness, eventually you will find that your Asana practice takes on a life of its own, flowing spontaneously into different postures according to your needs at the moment. Therefore, you should practice as taught by the Guru. If you want to evolve and reach perfection, then you have to practice according to the rules the Master has used and perfected for that process.

A Yogi should be free from anxiety with a steady mind to practice. Living in seclusion away from people in a place that is clean and a country that is well administered reduces the agitation of the mind. Insects, animals and other distractions should be eliminated. In other words, you have to be able to practice with focused intensity for the sole purpose of liberation, to reach the highest pinnacle of evolution. And to be able to practice with that kind of intensity, you have to reach a stage in your development where you are free from anxiety and wavering thoughts.

SIX CAUSES OF FAILURE

15
THE SIX CAUSES OF FAILURE IN YOGA ARE OVER-EATING, EXERTION, TALKATIVENESS, ADHERING TO RULES, WRONG ASSOCIATION AND RESTLESSNESS.

This is extremely important. If you find that you are practicing for many years and you are not improving, then examine your practice and see if any of these causes are violated.

Overeating

Overeating is one of the biggest obstacles that people face. It is ingrained in them from childhood when they first experienced indiscipline in diet. People continuously eat, following an instinct to survive, a Samskara that is very strong and inherited from our lower animal existence. In our lower existence, we had to struggle hard to get food to eat. Yet it is not in the nature of the lower species to overeat. They simply eat when they are hungry and stop when they are full. Nonetheless, they still have to struggle hard to get it.

When you reach the level of a human being, you have a mind and an intellect that can be used to acquire lots of food. You feel liberated and want to enjoy it. The problem arises because you continue enjoying it even when you have had enough.

Master Sivananda's first guideline concerning food is actually very simple and to the point: observe a moderate and balanced diet. Diet should never be complicated. He also suggested that we should eat only when we are hungry. The secret of good health is to be a little hungry all the time. Indigestion and congestion are the result of bad eating habits. The stomach is like a balloon. It expands if you eat too much. The next time you eat, that space will have to be filled again. You will find that when you eat less or after fasting, you are not able to consume as much anymore. That is because the stomach has shrunk.

If you overeat, what happens to you? You experience sluggishness. Tamas is one of the greatest obstacles to Sadhana. Overeating contributes a great deal to this. If you eat too much, you clog the bodily systems. Then toxins accumulate, thereby overtaxing and stressing the bodily systems, causing all the organs to work overtime, which in turn causes most of the food's energy to be expended in processing the food, assimilating it and eliminating the waste. That is why Master Sivananda said that you dig your grave with your teeth.

The body needs nourishment. But if it is already nourished, there is no need for more food. The body will either eliminate it or store it as fat. In the latter case, one will also need extra food to sustain the fat cells. Even body builders must eat to maintain that "extra" body. They form a habit of eating six to eight times a day. Such individuals become a slave to the body. Their mind is on food most of the time, which does not serve a higher purpose. It is a waste of energy, a waste of life, and a waste of God's gift.

It is through bad habits, bad eating, wrong understanding and wrong conditioning that you kill yourselve. When you eat moderately, you feel very light and the body's energy can be used for Sadhana. When you eat, do not overload the stomach. Fill it part with food, part with water and leave some space for God. This way you will not experience sluggishness.

Exertion

You want to devote all your time to Sadhana. If you exert the body too much, you will be tired and want to sleep. You will not have clarity and energy to continue with your Sadhana, which is your main focus in your life now as a Yogi living by yourself in solitude and in accordance with the Scriptures.

Some people approach Yoga as if they are performing vigorous gymnastics. When they are finished with a session, they are so exhausted that they want to sleep. In that case, you could see how it violates the rules of Yoga. That is one of the causes of lack of success on the path of enlightenment.

The way we do Asana in a Sampoorna Yoga class energizes the body. Master Sivananda said in his commentary on Yoga that when you are involved in vigorous exercises, the Prana flows outward. In the practice of Asana in the Sampoorna Yoga system, you will experience that the Prana moves inward to energize and heal the internal organs, the endocrine system, the nervous system and all the other systems of the body. After a session, you will feel more energized and invigorated to continue your Sadhana.

Talkativeness

Talkativeness is another obstacle and it is one of the most degrading habits of most people. Master Sivananda describes this condition as lingual diarrhea. You talk all the time and what do you talk about? Nothing. You are just gossiping and talking madness. It drains your energy, agitates the mind and keeps the mind vibrating on a very superficial level. You are not able to have that steadiness and strength of mind to probe into the deeper levels of self inquiry. So avoid too much long talk, tall talk, sweet talk, idle talk, etc.

What about the Yogi living in a hermitage in solitude? Can he be practicing talkativeness alone? Yes, because the mind can still be chattering. These instructions are for everybody even though we say it is for the Yogi. These are the laws of success and failure.

Talkativeness also means gathering all kinds of information, constantly reading various books, newspapers and magazines, as well as keeping up with the news. This is all talkativeness because the mind is chattering. Whereas for the Yogi who is living in solitude, why is he living there? To practice according to the instructions of the Guru. So he does not need to read so many different things. He will spend his time in the practice of Yoga. But people who are accustomed to socializing and gossiping, even when they are by themselves, will still need to read something, watch television, or listen to all sorts of things. It is a constant habit of distracting the mind.

Adhering to Rules

Be discriminative and flexible in order to devote most of your time to Sadhana. Eliminate the unnecessary rituals in which the average person squanders their time. Time is very precious and should not be wasted.

Sometimes it is necessary to follow rules but at other times, it is not important. When I get up in the morning, I quickly brush my teeth, wash my face and proceed swiftly to meditation because I do not want to waste that precious time. Especially when you are living by yourself, then you do not need to follow so many rules. You do not have to worry that you are offending other people. You do not have to follow any schedule. Therefore you can meditate as long as you want, chant as long and as loud as you want and wherever you want. You will never have to think about whether you may be disturbing other people. You eat when you are hungry, which means you can have breakfast at 1:00 or 2:00 p.m. There really are no rules. You just continue doing your Sadhana. Day and night are the same to you.

Swami Nada-Brahmananda told me that when he was doing Sadhana, he got up whenever he wanted, even if it was in the middle of the night or at 2:00 a.m. in the morning. He sang as long as he wanted, then went back to sleep, got up again, etc. There is no specific time to do anything. These rules do not apply to you anymore. You no longer think, "I must get up early in the morning at 6:00 a.m. for meditation. The bell rings so now I have to go for food."

You may also find that you have been following certain rules and conventions for so long that your mind has become very stuck and there is no room for exploration or discovering new things. I think that this is the dilemma everyone is facing today. They read a book that contains certain thoughts and ideas and they take it at face value, adopting it as their own, without the courage to question it or discern something different in it, like a seed that is planted and meant to grow. Everyone sees things through their own conditioning. Just because something is in a book or somebody comments on it does not necessarily mean that it is right or authoritative. That is what happened with the various commentaries on *Hatha Yoga Pradipika*. Everybody was commenting on Yoga by following the ideas of other commentators but no one had the courage to see it differently.

Wrong Association

Wrong association is one of the major causes of failure. As a spiritual aspirant, your path is outlined very clearly, and if you associate with people who are involved in your kind of discipline, then it will encourage and inspire you to evolve. But if you associate with people who are not interested in that, it will not encourage or help you, and it may even degrade your consciousness and destroy you.

For instance, if you associate with so-called intellectual people whose Guru might teach them something different from what you are doing, you might get into an argument about who is right and who is wrong, which is a useless activity.

Restlessness

Restlessness, or in other words, unsteadiness or a wavering and wandering mind, is another pitfall. What is the main cause of unsteadiness of the mind? Desires. The mind manufactures thoughts because of desires. How do you reach that desireless state? By first spiritualizing the desires, which is what the Yogi does by desiring enlightenment and liberation.

Desires that are based on selfishness, greed and lust, or prompted by egocentric wishes to satisfy the ego, the little self, will bind you and create negative Karma. It will create agitation in the mind.

Therefore, you could say that the primary sources of agitation or unsteadiness of the mind are lust, greed, hatred, jealousy, envy and fear. Lusting for power, wealth, name and fame, for example, are the things that create turbulence and extreme agitation in the mind. The process is to spiritualize your desires. Allow your desire to be for the highest, for God. That is why Saint Kabhir said, "Detach and attach!" Detach from the world and worldly thoughts and attach to God. That detachment from the world will only come when you see the imperfection in it, when you see the transient nature of it.

Sadhana is intense activity, intense self-effort. Nothing is achieved unless there is self-effort. To the extent you are exercising self-effort, that is the extent to which you are going to evolve, grow and transform. It is not a passive state. It is not a state where you do not do anything, just sitting and being lazy and useless all the time. People ask, "How long will it take to reach the goal?" This is foolish. Success will depend on how much effort you put in, not how much a Guru touches you. That is what most people think. If you touch them, they get Shaktipat and get enlightened. They do not even know what Shaktipat is. Success is in direct proportion to the effort you put in. But it is very important to be guided by right instruction. You can put in lots of self-effort, but if it is not directed in the right way, then you are wasting your time and effort. These are very important things to understand.

You have a certain goal that you want to achieve, but instead of pursuing that goal, you get distracted with other things, which dilute the strength and focus of the mind. That is why Master Sivananda said to practice stick-to-itiveness. Stick to it until the goal is reached. The nature of the mind is to procrastinate, to always put off until tomorrow what needs to be done today. Whatever you have to do now, the mind will always find something else to do instead. You convince yourself that you will attend to the initial task later. Maybe you have a month's time to complete it. But when the month is coming to a close and the project is not yet finished, it will create undue stress in your mind. By sticking to the task at hand, you develop strength of mind and your will becomes stronger. These are ways of disciplining the mind.

Lack of contentment or appreciation for the gifts and blessings that God has given you also leads to unsteadiness. Appreciate and enjoy what you have. When you "stop and smell the roses," your agitation will subside.

16
**THE SIX CAUSES OF SUCCESS IN YOGA ARE ENTHUSIASM, PERSEVER-
ANCE, RIGHT DISCRIMINATION, UNSHAKEABLE FAITH, COURAGE AND
RIGHT ASSOCIATION.**

These are the six causes of success not only in Yoga but in all endeavors.

Enthusiasm

As a practitioner, disciple and student, what is the first thing you must have?
Enthusiasm. If there is no enthusiasm, you are like a dead person. Imagine a dead
person sitting in front of a teacher. Nothing will flow from the teacher. The Guru
will ask, "What do you want? Do you want coffee?" You give them coffee, biscuits and blessings, and then they disappear. These people only have enthusiasm
for coffee, biscuits and blessings. But people who have enthusiasm and an intense
desire to learn and to transform themselves, will inspire the knowledge necessary
for spiritual growth to flow from the Guru. So you must have enthusiasm. That
is what will encourage or inspire the teacher to teach you. The teacher will know
that you are very enthusiastic to learn. It is the same thing with everybody. Take a
child for example. If the child is not enthusiastic, he will play with his toys alone
while the parents attend to their work without paying any attention to him. But
the moment the child jumps up enthusiastically to show his parents something,
evincing a genuine interest to learn, the parents become delighted and could
spend all day with the child.

Some people might appear to be enthusiastic at first but when you teach them,
you discover that you are really wasting your time because they only come to be

entertained. They are very enthusiastic but it is for entertainment value only. Many people attend lectures with a set amount of questions, asking every teacher and spiritual person the same exact questions. But the underlying motivation is really to impress the teacher and others with their nicely posed questions. They do not actually understand the answers or put them into practice because they are not genuinely interested in changing. Thus, sincere enthusiasm for learning is a very important quality of a student.

Perserverance

You have to put into practice what you have learned and persevere until the goal is reached. What is practice? As Maharishi Patanjali states in one of his Sutras, "Practice is the repeated effort to follow the disciplines which give permanent control of the thought waves of the mind." In other words, practice is repeated uninterrupted effort to gain mastery of what you have been taught.

Right Discrimination

There must also be right discrimination. You must cultivate the ability to have right discrimination. Do you know how much effort people put into stupidity? If you have been to college, you know what I am talking about. How much liquor can you hold? How many hotdogs and hamburgers can you eat at a time? How many cigarettes can you smoke? How long can you inhale? How long can you have sex? How many sexual partners can you have? And the list goes on. Imagine all the effort expended on such nonsensical things. People actually try to master these things! So you must have right discrimination. If there is no right discrimination, then you will waste your life in useless activity.

It is the same with everything. Even with singing and music, you can play music but what kind of music do you choose to play? You can put lots of self-effort into music that will degrade you. It is not going to elevate your consciousness. Look at a concert pianist, guitarist or a pop-artist. It takes so much effort to do what they do. But where is it leading them? To riches, fame, fortune, egocentricity, etc. It is not leading them to enlightenment. Now I am not saying that it is necessarily a bad thing. Through their achievements, they might have learned important qualities needed on the path to enlightenment, such as discipline to practice, self-effort, stick-to-itiveness and focus. But at a certain point, it is time to continue the journey or you will get stuck or even degrade your consciousness. This is even true with Asanas. Some people spend their entire life doing Asanas without moving beyond the physical aspect of Hatha Yoga practice. In that case, they have strayed from the path of Yoga.

Unshakeable Faith

You must also have unshakeable faith. Unshakeable faith in what? In the teachings of your Guru and the Scriptures. People have unshakeable faith in so many different things. You will persevere in whatever you have unshakeable faith in because you will be enthusiastic about it. Unless there is unshakeable faith, there is no intense enthusiasm. Without enthusiasm, you will not persevere in achieving something. When your interest is only half-hearted, you think, "Oh, I'll see how it works and then . . . ." And then you leave it at that.

Courage

Without courage, you lack the boldness you need to persevere because as soon as you encounter any kind of obstacle, hardship or doubt, you just give up and take the easy way out. You do not have the courage to dare to continue. As soon as your body hurts a little, you give up. Yet people persevere so much in things that are very degrading and damaging. Some people snort cocaine even though they know it destroys the brain. But if you ask the same people to do some Yoga, they are afraid that they might pull a muscle, or even worse, die. People study all the contraindications. They believe it must be very comfortable. Therefore, they conclude that the way to practice Yoga should be easy. They do Yoga for years but they do not improve. They use words like "non-violence" and then justify practicing non-violence in their Yoga. They never go beyond what feels comfortable because they lack courage to go beyond the limits they have established for themselves. This stunts their growth on all levels.

You must have courage to really dare to explore. Spiritual practice is exploring into the unknown: that which you do not know, cannot see, cannot hear, etc. Yet you have the faith and the desire to improve and free yourself from all the addictions, conditioning and limitations. And then you see your Guru who has done it and who knows the way, so you have the unshakeable faith in your Guru, the Scriptures and all the Rishis who tell you about the glories of God-realization, the glories of gaining control of your mind, your senses, your emotions, etc. But you must have courage.

Once I was convinced about the path of Yoga, I felt many odd sensations while practicing, including feeling as if my hand was paralyzed. Yet I had the courage to continue. I had pinched a nerve but I did not realize it at the time. Now I am not recommending that you do not listen to the warning signs of your body. But at the time I was experiencing this, I did not care if I died doing Yoga. People die doing so many things, including taking drugs such as cocaine, angel dust, ecstasy, etc., even though they see the adverse effects. Notwithstanding the fact that they see other people dying from drug abuse, they are convinced it will be different for them. This is sheer foolishness. On the other hand, you have never seen anybody drop dead doing Yoga!

Some people's bodies are in such a toxic condition that any kind of movement will trigger muscles spasms. So why would it be different with Yoga? The moment they make a movement and feel anything other than peace, they blame Yoga. It is not Yoga's fault. It is the condition of the body. So you must have courage.

Right Association

Avoid the company of common people. This means to avoid wrong association and seek right association! We talked about this in the last Sloka. The association must be in harmony with the path that you are following. It can also apply to the books you read, the movies that you see, the music that you listen to, etc. This is all association. If you examine these things properly, you can see how important it is for success in life and success in your Sadhana.

To Summarize:

For the spiritual aspirant, right association means to be in the company of seekers of Truth or God. This will inspire right discrimination and prompt you to pursue the true goal and purpose of life, which is enlightenment. Such a noble aspiration will mystically lead you to your Guru. In the beginning, however, there will be doubts as to whether the Guru you are following is right for you and capable of guiding you to your goal. This is where right discrimination will help you. You will have unshakeable faith in your Guru and his teachings when you are convinced that his teachings correspond to those of the Scriptures and the Masters, that they are logical and reasonable, and that he himself lives what he teaches and you can see the positive results of his practice in his own life. This unshakable faith is extremely important in order to persevere in your Sadhana with intense enthusiasm. As you persevere, you will no doubt encounter many obstacles to overcome because the spiritual path is paved with innumerable roadblocks. The most prominent obstacles are the six causes of failure which you must fervently guard against. Family and old friends who are immersed in the world and do not aspire for liberation will undoubtedly try to discourage you and break your faith under the misguided pretense that they care for you and your welfare. That is when right discrimination will prove to be your real friend. You will know whole-heartedly that your Guruís teaching and guidance is true. This will give you the courage to pursue your Sadhana until the goal is reached.

YAMAS

17

THE TEN YAMAS IN HATHA YOGA ARE NON-INJURY, NON-LYING, NON-STEALING, CONTINENCE, FORGIVENESS, ENDURANCE, COMPASSION, HUMILITY, MODERATE DIET AND CLEANLINESS.

In Hatha Yoga, there are ten Yamas, rules of moral conduct, and ten Niyamas, ethical observances, whereas in Raja Yoga, there are five Yamas and five Niyamas. Here, it is broken down into more basic forms so that you can deepen your understanding. The five Yamas and Niyamas in the Raja Yoga system are not deficient because there are fewer of them. Rather they are more condensed.

In Raja Yoga, the five Yamas are non-injury, non-lying, non-stealing, non-covetousness and sexual purity.

Non-Injury and Non-Lying

In a more advanced stage of understanding, non-injury includes refraining from creating harm to any creature in thoughts, words and deeds. Truthfulness implies not telling a lie under any circumstance. When should you speak the truth if you should refrain from creating harm to anyone in words? If you know that speaking the truth is going to cause harm to someone, then you remain quiet. For example, if a murderer enters your house chasing someone who hides in your closet and then asks you where he went, you should not tell him the truth because he is going to kill that person. In that case, you should remain silent. If you knowingly try to hurt someone with the truth, you are creating violence. Now that does not mean that you should never tell the truth if you know someone's feelings may be hurt. For example, a Guru is going to be as straightforward as possible because he is trying to teach his disciples, even if it impinges on their ego. Sometimes students will react emotionally but they need to wake up to the truth and face reality. That is not considered hurting someone with words. In fact, the Guru is actually helping the disciple.

Non-Stealing

Non-stealing means do not covet what other people have and do not take what is not yours. In a deeper sense, it connotes that if you have more than you need, then you are stealing from the rest of humanity.

Continence

Continence or Brahmacharya is moderation in all sensual pleasures and not just abstinance from sex. However, you do not need to indulge in sexual pleasures for survival. Instead, this energy can be sublimated to accelerate your evolution.

Yoga is a means to take you to the point of transcendence, where you are able to have direct experience of the Divine Self. This takes place when the mind becomes calm, steady and peaceful like a lake. We need our senses to function in this world and that is why God gave them to us. The senses help us to be efficient when they function properly. However, if these senses are stimulated excessively, then the mind becomes weak and fragmented. The mind actually moves outward through the senses so that the more the senses are stimulated, the more fragmented and weaker the mind becomes. That is why Brahmacharya is really disciplining of the senses. It is not just curtailing sexual activity. Because people misunderstand this, they mistakenly think that Brahmacharya is just suppressing sexual activity. Then they indulge in other aspects of sensual pleasure, like overeating, which also dissipates their energy and creates many health problems. By living a life of discipline, you will enjoy good health and peace of mind.

Now let us examine sexual activity. If you do not have sex, you are not going to die because you do not need it to survive. In other words, this energy can be conserved and directed towards your Sadhana. In many religious institutions, observance of celibacy is a rule or regulation that must be obeyed. More often than not, the people following such rules are not informed as to the reason for celibacy or how to sublimate the energy for Sadhana. All they know is that it is a law or rule of the church. In Yoga, you are not actually suppressing sexual activity. You learn to sublimate it or engage in it moderately. If you do not express it and you do not know how to sublimate it, then it is likely that you are going to suffer all kinds of problems such as stress, anxiety and emotional turmoil.

It is you who wants to be in control of your mind. It is not something that is imposed on you. You become aware that your mind and emotions are ruling you and driving you crazy. Yet you know that you are capable of more. Thus, you seek ways to gain control of the mind.

In the study and practice of Yoga, you observe celibacy. But this is not just confined to Yoga. For example, if a boxer wants to win a world championship in boxing, his coaches will instruct him to live a disciplined life, to exercise and to refrain from sexual activity for a period of time during training. Now why would a boxer be instructed to refrain from sex? If it was not affecting his stamina and focus, his coaches would not impose it. The boxer who wants to win will observe these rules. It is the same thing with Yoga. All the Masters tell you that if you want to gain control of your mind and reach the state of transcendence, there are certain rules and laws that need to be followed. Moderation in sexual pleasures is one of them. It is not that they have anything against sex. But they know that by involving yourself in it, you are dissipating your energy uselessly.

How would you dissipate your energy in sexual activity? For example, when you are engaged in sex and enjoy it, what happens? You become attached to each other, especially the person who enjoyed it more. In fact, you might want to possess and own each other. If the other person is of a lower consciousness, he or she will try to pull you down to their level to feel comfortable. Very rarely will that person try to uplift their consciousness to your level. Thus, you can see how you are involved not just on a physical level, but on an emotional level and with consciousness itself. As a result, the act of sex is now creating disturbance in your mind.

In contrast, two Yogis of the same level and consciousness can enjoy sex because it will be done without attachment or emotional entanglement. When you want to enjoy something and do it without any kind of trauma or attachment, then it does not lead to addiction. You see it for what it is. You enjoy it but you do not get attached to it. If you do not get it tomorrow, you will not crave it. Thus, you will not be dissipating your energy. In the example given above, the Yogis would be practicing Tantric Yoga, which is discussed more fully in Chapter 3 in relation to Vajroli Mudra. But in order to have reached that state, they must have been observing Yamas and Niyamas and evolved their consciousness to a high state.

Approaching this from another perspective, when you eat your food, that food is digested and processed to build the Dhatus, which are the different cells in your body. These are Rasa, plasma; Rakta, blood; Mamsa, muscle; Meda, fat; Asti, bone; Majja, marrow and nerves; and Shukra and Artav, reproductive tissue. Food is first turned into plasma and then it is further distilled into blood and so on until the end product becomes Shukra Dhatu or the reproductive cells, which is the subtlest essence of the digestive process of food. Master Sivananda, who was a medical doctor and a great spiritual Master, said that the body takes about 13 days distilling the food and storing the subtlest essence to fill the cup of sexual energy. That is why normally, after a certain time of the month, people who do not indulge in sex excessively, will suddenly feel sexual urges. When that happens, they will want to be with their partner. If you express this sexual energy, the cup is empty, so to speak, and then the body starts to distill the Shukra Dhatu again. This cycle continues throughout your lifetime as a normal human being. You grow up, get old and eventually die.

The Yogis have found that this does not necessarily have to be the end product of that energy. They discovered that it can be sublimated from Shukra Dhatu into Ojas Shakti (mental energy) Tejas and Prana. When this sexual energy is sublimated, it becomes mental energy, which means that your mind becomes very fertile. Your retentive power will increase and you will experience more steadiness. On the other hand, if you observe people who engage in sexual activity often, they are usually very agitated. It is dissipating their energy and scattering their mind. Their attention is diverted elsewhere. When this energy is sublimated, it becomes Ojas Shakti and Tejas. You can actually see brilliance in the person's face. He or she will exude a certain radiance. The Prana, which is really the actual life force, is also enhanced and increased. Therefore they will have pranic power and mental clarity.

When you stay at an Ashram, abstinence from sexual activity is not the only reason your energy is enhanced. The mind is in a Sattwic state because you become involved in positive activity and positive thoughts. You eat pure food that is not exciting sexual thoughts and sexual hormones. Then you can experience the different level in your thinking power, your mental power, the way you behave and the way you act. You can see for yourself how your energy is increased.

Now, I am not advising that you should never have sexual activity, particularly if you are married. Do not think of this as a problem or else it becomes a suppression. If you are married and you feel that you want to express your love, sex will not be a mechanical thing. It will only be an expression of your love. And if it is expressed in that way, it becomes something very beautiful and very fulfilling. You will even find that you get a lot of energy from it if it is done with right understanding and as an expression of love. However, you will discover that as you continue your Sadhana, the urge to express your love sexually becomes less and less. The reality is that sex is often only by force of habit. You probably feel that your partner wants to have sex tonight, and so you may instigate it. At the same time, your partner is probably feeling that you probably want to have sex. If there is sincerity, honesty and communication between you, you can be forthright with your desires or lack of desires. Then you will discover that just being with each other is more blissful and fulfilling.

In a marriage, both persons should feel equally important to contribute to each other's welfare, well-being and happiness. If that is the case, then there will be joyfulness. And if both of you feel that you want to express your love sexually, then express it without any reservation or inhibition. If you find that the other person is having a problem with it in the form of an addiction, try to help that person. In any kind of sensual activity, there is the possibility of becoming addicted. Pleasure can lead to addiction. Therefore, you can help them through love and understanding. Help them understand that there is a higher way.

There are certain things that may stimulate certain desires or urges in society. That is why Satsanga, right association, is important. If you are in association with people that are not encouraging or thinking about sexual activity, then you are not activating or stimulating your sexual glands or thoughts. Sex is really thoughts. If your mind is not there, then it is not initiating it. Food and diet are very important. Eat moderately and refrain from eating things that are stimulating like garlic, onion and spices. You should also avoid foods known to be aphrodisiacs, which stimulate sexual activity.

Even though some of the Scriptures and Masters have admonished that you should completely avoid women and not even look at them, this is ignorance and a very negative way of thinking. Look at women as divine, as if they were your mother or your sister. Women are a manifestation of divinity. They personify beauty, tenderness, softness, love, compassion and essence. If you look at every woman with sexual thoughts, then it is your problem. It is not the problem of the women. Try to cultivate divine vision. Divinity exists in every aspect of creation. From ancient times, the Gurus and Rishis were all married. Their relationship with their wife was just a manifestation of their counterpart. They were not whole without the other. You can see this with Vishnu and Lakshmi, Shiva and Shakti, and Brahma and Saraswati. There is always this interrelationship. There is not one without the other. Every aspect of nature is expressing this same divine relationship between the feminine and masculine. The feminine aspect is beauty, softness and essence.

Some people are constantly looking for their other half to be complete and are miserable when they cannot find it. That is because they really do not understand or know the purpose of the counterpart. A relationship with another person can help you to reach the real beloved, which is God, your true Self. In Yoga, we say that Shakti separates from Shiva. Because of this separation, we feel empty, deficient and less than whole. Therefore we look for this wholeness and completeness in relationships. Through right understanding and proper relationship, you can experience something divine, full and complete.

Now, if you are experiencing something from a higher level of completeness and fullness, then there is nothing deficient in you. You do not need relationships. You do not need things. You do not need disciples. You do not need anything. In that case, you are naturally going to be observing moderation of the senses.

Forgiveness

The next Yama, forgiveness, comes into play when you feel that somebody has done something wrong to you and you hold malice, a grudge, hatred or you want revenge. All these things arise from not being able to forgive. By not letting go and holding onto these things, you create more poison, disease and turbulence in your own mind. You are not actually doing anything to the other person. That person is long gone and has left you alone with your trauma and poison. You are only torturing yourself. So why not forgive?

Endurance

Endurance is essential on the spiritual path. Once you have made the resolve to do Sadhana, it demands a great deal of endurance. Some people give up as soon as they feel a little discomfort. When you first start doing Sadhana like Asana and Pranayama, you begin purifying your body and might experience a lot of pain and discomfort. Remember, it is a process to reverse your outgoing nature and your indiscipline. It takes energy, strength, courage and effort. Do not give up.

Compassion

Compassion is necessary. If you do not have compassion, you will be irritated constantly. You may see someone suffering and just turn a blind eye or walk the other way. Whatever you send out into the world comes back to you for learning. If you try to cultivate these qualities within yourself, it will help to purify your own mind and to release you from hatred, jealousy, envy, etc.

Humility

Humility is another vow. If you do not have humility, then you will not have compassion. You will feel that you are greater than everybody else and you will not be tolerant or compassionate. Humility is necessary to help you reduce your ego. If you do not have humility, then your ego becomes more magnified. Humility is a measure of readiness for higher evolution. It dissolves the cocoon of negative conditioning and makes you ready and receptive for the Guru to pour knowledge into you.

Moderate diet

Moderate diet is one of the rules of success. Moderate diet means that you should not overload your stomach by eating too much. Overeating will burden the digestive system and hampers digestion, assimilation and elimination. This will create lots of toxins and poisons in your body, resulting in sickness and a great deal of uneasiness. The end result is that you will not be able to meditate or do Sadhana.

Cleanliness

Cleanliness means you should be clean in thoughts, words and deeds. Cleanliness is next to Godliness. It helps you to establish the state of Sattwa in your mind and personality. A person who does not wash himself, bathe his skin or brush his teeth, becomes a menace to society. If you come to Satsang like that, everybody will run away from you because you will be distracting and disturbing them. Even outward cleanliness is a practice that helps to move towards Sattwa, the state of purity. This includes not wearing perfumes, hairspray or deoderants that disturb the sense of smell in others, particularly Yogis and Gurus who are very sensitive to odors.

The Yamas are like resolves you make. You want to embody these qualities. Desire to be truthful and non-violent. Aspire to develop these qualities in your personality. These are your aspirations and true wealth. Now, how do you aquire these? Through the ten Niyamas.

18

THE TEN NIYAMAS ARE TAPAS, DANA, CONTENTMENT, BELIEF IN GOD, WORSHIP OF GOD, JAPA, LISTENING AND STUDY OF THE SCRIPTURES, MODESTY, A DISCERNING INTELLECT AND YAJNA.

These are the ten Niyamas or practices that will help you to acquire the qualities called Yamas.

Tapas

This means living a life of discipline which helps to keep balance in the individual. This is obtained through the different components of Sadhana, or spiritual practices, Yoga postures, breathing exercises, meditation, proper diet, positive thinking, good company and study of the Scriptures.

To promote the sattvic quality in the individual, the Scriptures prescribe austerity of body, speech and mind to be practiced in this manner: a.) To worship God, have reverence for the Seers, Sages and Gurus, and to practice straightforwardness, non-injury and celebacy are called austerity of the body. b.) To speak pleasantly, truthfully and beneficially without hurting others and to study the Scriptures regularly is austerity of speech. c.) To practice serenity, sympathy, silence, self-control and purity of motive is called austerity of mind.

Dana

Practicing charity is to free oneself from selfishness and greed, which are great obstacles to enlightenment. It is acknowledging our social responsibility towards our family, our community and our country, recognizing that we are citizens of the world. This is done not only through the payment of taxes but also in contributing to charitable work and in supporting Ashrams, Sanyasins, etc. according to one's means. Dana helps to maintain balance in society.

Contentment

Contentment is a necessary practice, otherwise you will constantly be hankering after everything and seeking what everybody else has. Without contentment, you are involved in the rat race and you may not appreciate your parents, teachers, wife, husband, children or friends.

You may think that if you are always content with what you have, then you do not progress much because you will be satisfied with where you are now. However, if you do not appreciate what you have, your mind is constantly agitated, thinking that the grass is greener on the other side. You believe that you must acquire more things to become happy. But if you appreciate what you have, then you can enjoy it and still strive for greater attainment. Because most people do not appreciate what they have, they lack confidence and always feel inadequate. On a physical level, no matter how much people possess, since they are not content, they always feel the need for something else to make them happy. They never appreciate or enjoy what they already have. This is true on all levels: physical, emotional, mental and intellectual.

Stop and smell the roses! Learn to appreciate what you have. Be thankful and grateful for it. This does not mean that you get stuck there. If you have the capacity and desire to achieve more, then do it. You could say that the inability to be content is an expression of ungratefulness. Contentment does not handicap you. In fact, it creates the condition for greater achievement when you appreciate and work with what you have. If some people do not get what they consider to be the appropriate, expected or correct tool to perform a specified task, they are suddenly unable to do the work. They cannot improvise. They lack contentment. With contentment comes ingenuity and creativity. Contentment is not a tamasic resignation. It is more akin to appreciation.

There is an old adage about a man with no shoes. The man cried that he did not have shoes. Then one day he was walking down the street and saw another man who did not have feet. That made him feel ashamed. "My God, I still have feet. Hallelujah! Praise the Lord! Thank you God!" That is contentment.

On a deeper level, contentment means that you stop searching for happiness and fullness outside in the material world or in other people. It brings your attention to what is here now in your life and even turns your focus inward, toward the Self, to realize your fullness.

Belief in God and Worship of God

Next, you must have belief and faith in the Supreme God, in the teachings of your Guru and in the Scriptures. Again, this is unshakeable faith. You must also worship God through rituals, prayers, chanting, singing, Puja and Satsanga. Listening to the recitations of sacred Scriptures and discourses on God All these things help to purify the mind and keep it in a Sattwic, positive and divine state.

Japa

Japa or Mantra repetition is a way to develop constant remembrance of God. It is also one of the most efficient and positive way to develop concentration of mind and get rid of its impurities. In much the same way as one cleans a vessel by continuously pouring clean water in it until all the impurities have flowed out, Mantra repetition takes away all the impurities of the mind and drowns out its noise. Eventually, only the divine vibration will remain. The Mantra will be so rooted in the mind that it will stay in the background day and night. It essentially impregnates the mind with the divine name. That is the purpose of the practice. Contact is made with the specific manifestation of God or Ishta Devata (chosen ideal). As God's power abides in his name, the Mantra becomes a constant support and protection. It transforms the personality in subtle ways and brings true happiness. Japa is first done aloud. After awhile, as one becomes more in tune with the subtler vibrations, the repetition becomes increasingly more internalized. This leads to the transcendental state until eventually it connects with the source.

Listening and Studying the Scriptures:

Satsanga means to associate with seekers of self-knowledge. This is why, whenever you have the opportunity to be in the company of enlightened beings, you should take advantage of it. In the absence of that facility, studying the Scriptures is the next best thing. Even better is to study the Scriptures with your Guru, because if you study on your own, you may understand quite the opposite of what is meant. Scriptures can be interpreted on seven levels and only a Guru with deep insight and intuition can reveal the truth to you. He understands the various levels of the teachings and will explain it in a manner that befits your level of consciousness. Listening to the explanations your Guru gives on the Scriptures will increase your devotion to God and inspire you to continue your Sadhana for the goal of liberation. This is the best association you can have. Discourse on the Scriptures from a Guru is, in essence, connection with enlightened Rishis who have experienced absolute truth. Because of their unconditional love and desire to alleviate the suffering of humanity, these Rishis put their experience in writing to serve as a map for struggling and sincere aspirants and to steer them away from the innumerable pitfalls ahead in their Sadhana.

Modesty

Modesty is an expression of humility and refinement. A cultured person will dress appropriately according to the occasion. Modesty also means not to show off and demonstrate your knowledge and powers to others but to be humble.

Discerning intellect

This means you should cultivate right discrimination, as explained earlier under the six causes of success in Sadhana.

Yajna

This means sacrifice, which is acknowledging the omnipresence of the Divine and knowing that your sustenance comes from God. This practice develops a reverence and a gratitude that will naturally be reflected in respect and care for nature. Worship, devotion, rituals and prayers are other means of expressing gratitude and connecting with the Divine. The ancients recognized that behind every aspect of nature, there is a presiding "Devata" that needs to be nourished. Taking without giving anything back in return is equivalent to thievery. Therefore, a portion of the harvest was given in charity and in sacrificial fires. We know from our experience that if we take fruit from a tree without watering it and caring for it, its yield will diminish. So Yajna helps to establish balance in nature. Nowadays, we selfishly have a tendency to extract from nature everything it can give without paying attention to the consequences. That is why there are so many environmental disasters.

On another level, sacrifice means to be able to give up negative tendencies. To relinquish material things that are the source of your greed and selfishness. This whole universe is based on sacrifice. To be able to get something, you have to give up something. Nothing is for nothing. If you do not have a discerning intellect and are not careful, you will discover that you sacrifice things that are important to you for things which are not so important. Without right discrimination, you might give up your inheritance for a bowl of soup.

There is a classic story in the Bible. It is the story of two brothers, Isaak and Jakob. One day, Isaak arrived very hungry and asked his brother Jakob for a bowl of soup. Jakob, negotiated that Isaak had to trade his inheritance for the bowl of soup. Without thinking, Isaak agreed and ate the bowl of soup. When it was time for their father to divide his property to them, Jakob said to Isaak: "You have already forfeited your inheritance!"

To some people, this is just a story. But it has a very deep spiritual meaning and mystical implication. The essence of the story captures the nature of the world. People who are in a state of unawareness and desperation do not think and can be easily exploited. In one moment of indiscretion, one moment of not thinking or losing your discriminative faculty, you can trade your whole life for something that is very insignificant. One moment of pleasure can ruin your entire life. You take drugs and get AIDS, or you become addicted, or you have sex with some-body and it changes your whole life. It is so easy to slide down to hell.

So you have to be very vigilant as a spiritual aspirant, because to get something, you have to give something. That is the law of the universe. Always make sure that what you are getting is more valuable than what you are giving. This does not mean that you are stealing from somebody.

If you want to gain wisdom, you have to sacrifice your ignorance. People cling to their stupidity but still want to appear to be wise. It is very simple. If you want to be healthy, you have to sacrifice your sickness. If you want to have strength of mind, you have to sacrifice your weakness and indiscipline. If you want liberation, you have to sacrifice your agitation of mind. That is why Jesus advised that you cannot serve God and Mammon at the same time. You cannot want to hold on to the world and still reach God. Practice detaching and attaching. Detach from the world and attach to God or your Ideal. That is sacrifice. Through sacrifice, you also create balance in society, nature and the individual.

These rules and laws are given here in the very beginning because they are the foundation for higher transformation. It does not mean that you have to be established in all this before you start Asana, but at least be aware of them and understand their importance since they are the foundation of any meaningful practice that will further your evolution. Understand the importance of right conduct and right aspiration. Understand the things that will destroy your success and the things that will bring success. Understand that the goal and the objective of your practice is to reach God, to reach perfection, to reach the highest state of evolution, referred to as Raja Yoga. Once this is clear in your mind, as you continue with your practice, Asanas and Pranayama, you will discover how it all fits into that grand scheme, that grand objective, and you will not get stuck in the superficial aspects of Asana practice.

Yamas and Niyamas are an essential part of spiritual practice. Whatever practice you are involved in, try to observe Yamas and Niyamas so that you can eradicate negative thoughts. When the mind is worry-free, you will have a greater capacity to do Sadhana.

You do not need to strive really hard to reach this. Just see the wisdom of it: observe how it frees you from your own enslavement and your own hell. Understand what these negative qualities, such as hatefulness, the inability to forgive, jealousy, etc., do to your mind! It imprisons and enslaves you, keeping you in hell. Now, do you want to free yourself? It is only you who will free yourself. If you continue to steal, cheat, lie and hurt other people, maybe the police will come to free you from that hell by locking you up in jail.

To be able to speak the truth, to be straightforward and honest is the most liberating thing. Only cowards do not want to be truthful. People think that if they are truthful, they are going to hurt somone. If the truth hurts you, then you have a big problem. It does not mean that you have to feed someone lies all the time. If you do, it shows that you do not have any strength or courage to speak the truth. Then you are violating the basic laws of success. It is better to be straightforward and honest because it creates steadiness in your own mind. Truth should not violate logic or reasoning and it should not transgress the Scriptures or the experience of enlightened Masters.

These rules are Kriyas for the mind. In other words, they purify the mind. If you examine them, you can see how important they are if you want to free the mind of its defects. What does purification of the mind actually mean? It means reducing the stress, agitation, restlessness and trauma of the mind. When that mind is traumatic, agitated, restless and contaminated by all kinds of negative feelings and thoughts, it is unfit for any kind of attainment, especially spiritual attainment. In fact, in such a state, it is not fit for anything.

That is what Yoga is all about. It serves to correct the defects of the mind and remove the impurities so that the mind can be steady, calm and peaceful, and regain its power to probe into the depths and the mysteries of life, such as: "Who am I?" Then the mind will be fit to know the Self, the Truth or God. It is only people who are endowed with this foundation that will have the aspiration and be fit to live in solitude to continue Sadhana for liberation.

A S A N A S

19

THE FIRST DISCIPLINE IN HATHA YOGA IS THE PRACTICE OF ASANA. THIS REFINES THE BODY RESULTING IN GOOD HEALTH AND STEADINESS.

Many commentators interpret this Sloka to mean that Asana comes first, prior to everything else, including Yama and Niyama. But these are practices that you are already now doing on the path of Hatha Yoga.

Just as with the first Sloka, this Sloka is the source of much confusion for commentators and teachers, who many in the world regard as genuine Hatha Yoga Masters. Putting aside the purpose of *Hatha Yoga Pradipika* and taking this Sloka out of context, one can say that Asana practice is an appropriate starting place for most people who want to start the practice of Yoga. From this perspective, many teachers keep people practicing Asana for years without any thought of introducing Yamas, Niyamas or breathing exercises.

Even if one is just starting out down the path of Hatha Yoga for health reasons, incorporating the five principles of proper exercise (Asana), proper breathing, proper relaxation, proper diet and positive thinking (as taught by my Guru, Swami Vishnudevananda), will greatly accelerate the healing process. Focusing on Asana alone is a precious waste of time and life, when this same time can be most profitably used by incorporating breathing exercises, relaxation techniques, awareness of proper diet and positive thinking (Yamas and Niyamas) into your practice as taught in Sampoorna Hatha Yoga. This approach tremendously enhances and accelerates the progress of the practitioner.

This Scripture is meant for someone who is ready for this stage of intensive Sadhana, as discussed earlier. Such a person is already a Hatha Yoga practitioner established in Dharma. So what is this Sloka referring to? It means that you continue your practice of Asana in a more intense manner to complete the refinement process of the physical systems so that good health is maintained and steadiness of the body is increased. In this way, the body will not be a distraction for the more advanced practices of Kumbhakas, Bandhas and Mudras. This fact is evident as the descriptions of Asanas given here are not meant for the beginner.

20
DESCRIBED HERE ARE SOME OF THE ASANAS THAT WERE TAUGHT BY SAGES LIKE VASHISHTHA AND YOGIS LIKE MATSYENDRANATH.

What follows next are some of the Asanas. According to the Scriptures, there are 84,000 postures, which probably indicates that there are infinite possibilities of Asanas. Essentially, every position and every movement is an Asana.

In the context of someone reaching the stage in his life where he is withdrawing from the world and dedicating all his time to Hatha Yoga Sadhana, he must have been practicing Yoga for some time where he has attained a high level of proficiency in Asana. We are not talking about someone who is first being introduced to Yoga and must approach Asana practice from a very basic level and then continue in a systematic manner to gain flexibility and comfort in the body. As you will observe, no beginner will be able to get into the postures described hereafter.

Some of the Asanas that are useful and important to the dedicated Sadhaka are described here. These are accepted by Munis like Vashishta and Yogis like Matsyendranath. Matsyendranath is supposed to be the first recipient of this knowledge from Shiva himself.

SWASTIKASANA

Auspicious Pose

21

PLACING THE SOLES OF BOTH FEET ON THE INNER THIGHS, SITTING FIRMLY WITH THE BODY ERECT, THIS IS CALLED SWASTIKASANA.

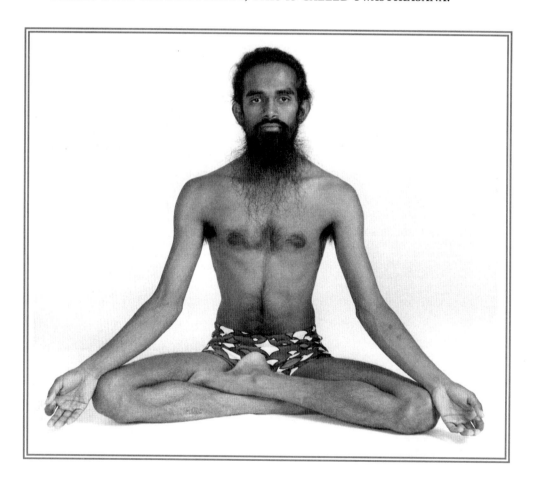

GOMUKHASANA

Cow's Face Pose

22

PLACE THE RIGHT ANKLE BY THE SIDE OF THE LEFT HIP AND THE LEFT ANKLE BY THE SIDE OF THE RIGHT HIP. THIS RESEMBLES THE FACE OF A COW AND IS CALLED GOMUKHASANA.

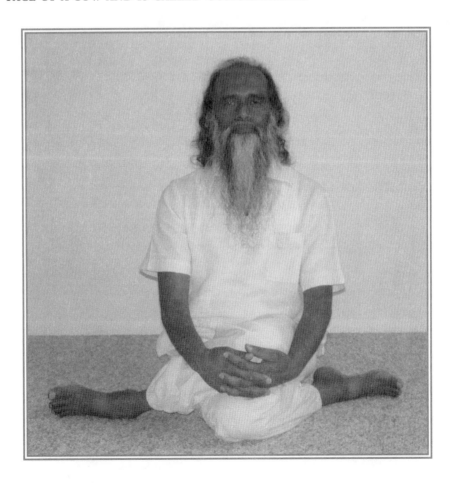

VIRASANA
Hero's Pose

23

PLACE ONE FOOT BY THE OPPOSITE THIGH AND THE OTHER FOOT UNDER THE SAME THIGH. THIS IS VIRASANA.

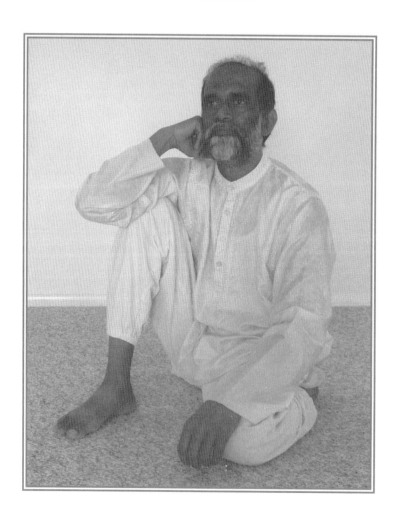

Kurmasana

Tortoise Pose

24
**PRESS FIRMLY THE LEFT SIDE OF THE ANUS WITH THE RIGHT ANKLE
AND THE RIGHT SIDE WITH THE LEFT ANKLE AND SIT WELL-POISED.
THIS IS KURMASANA ACCORDING TO THE YOGIS.**

If you try to do Kurmasana according to this Sloka, you will only experience pain.

The way my Guru taught me is to sit with the legs apart. Bend the knees slightly and slide the arms under the legs. Press the arms down with the legs as you bring the forehead or chin to the floor. In the more advanced stage, you can continue to bring the legs together until they cross over the head.

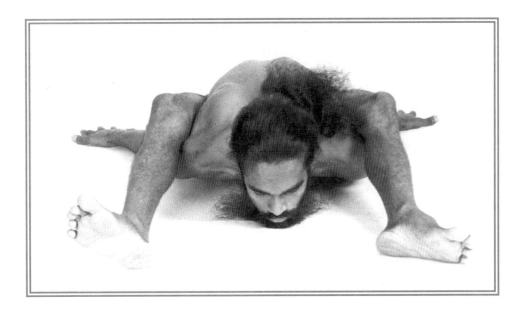

KUKKUTASANA
Rooster Pose

25

IN PADMASANA, INSERT THE ARMS BETWEEN THE CALVES AND THIGHS AND PLACING THE PALMS FIRMLY ON THE GROUND, PUSH THE BODY UP. THIS IS KUKKUTASANA.

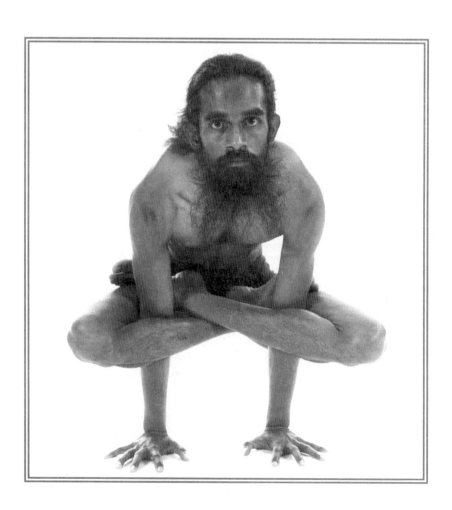

UTTANAKURMASANA
Stretching Tortoise Pose

26

IN PADMASANA, INSERT THE ARMS BETWEEN THE CALVES AND THIGHS AND INTERLACE THE FINGERS BEHIND THE NECK WHILE LYING ON THE BACK LIKE A TORTOISE. THIS IS UTTANAKURMASANA.

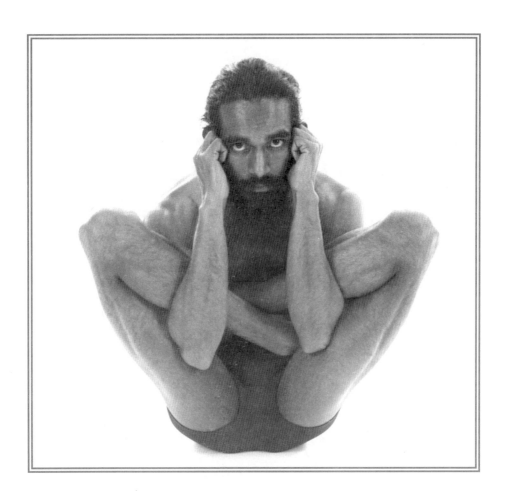

D H A N U R A S A N A

B o w   P o s e

27

LIE ON THE TUMMY AND BEND THE KNEES. REACH BACK AND GRAB
HOLD OF THE TOES AND PULL THEM TO THE EARS AS IF STRINGING A
BOW. THIS IS DHANURASANA.

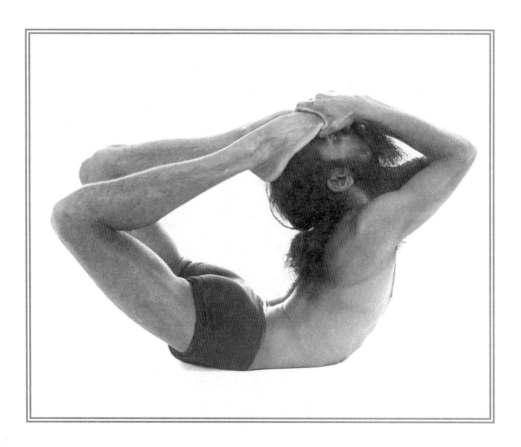

M A T S Y E N D R A S A N A
Spinal Twist

28

PLACE THE RIGHT FOOT AT THE ROOT OF THE LEFT THIGH AND THE LEFT FOOT AT THE OUTSIDE OF THE RIGHT KNEE. WIND THE RIGHT ARM AROUND THE LEFT KNEE AND GRAB HOLD OF THE LEFT FOOT. WIND THE LEFT ARM BEHIND THE WAIST AND TWIST TO THE LEFT. THIS ASANA IS NAMED AFTER SRI MATSYENDRANATH.

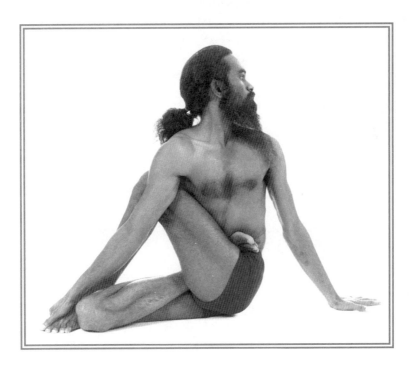

29

THE PRACTICE OF MATSYENDRASANA STIMULATES THE GASTRIC FIRE IN THE STOMACH AND IS A WEAPON THAT DESTROYS A NUMBER OF TERRIBLE DISEASES. IT AROUSES KUNDALINI SHAKTI AND STABILIZES THE BINDU.

PASCHIMOTTANASANA
Forward Bend Pose

30

STRETCH THE LEGS IN FRONT ON THE GROUND LIKE STICKS AND
BENDING FORWARD, HOLD THE TOES WITH BOTH HANDS AND PLACE
THE FOREHEAD ON THE KNEES. THIS IS PASCHIMOTTANASANA.

31

PASCHIMOTTANASANA IS VERY BENEFICIAL. IT CAUSES THE PRANIC
CURRENT TO FLOW THROUGH SUSHUMNA, INCREASES THE GASTRIC
FIRE, FLATTENS THE ABDOMEN AND BESTOWS GOOD HEALTH.

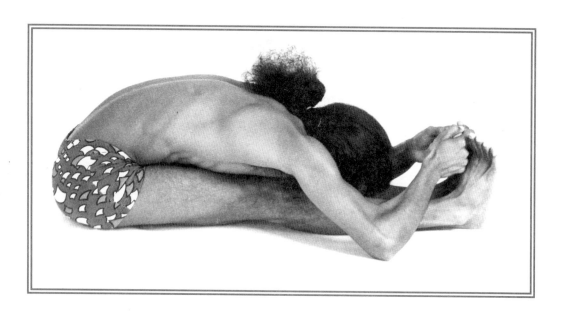

MAYURASANA

Peacock Pose

32
**PLACE THE PALMS ON THE GROUND. BRING THE ELBOWS TOGETHER
AND PLACE THEM ON BOTH SIDES OF THE NAVEL. STRETCH THE BODY
HORIZONTALLY LIKE A STICK AND BALANCE IN THE AIR. THIS IS
MAYURASANA.**

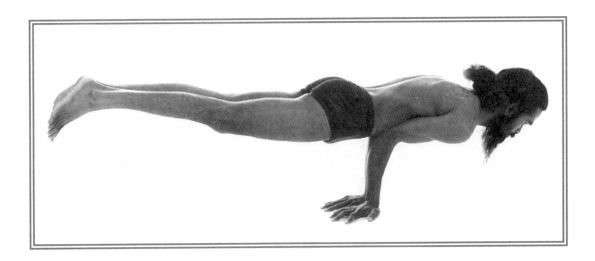

33

MAYURASANA SOON DESTROYS ALL DISEASES OF THE SPLEEN AND STOMACH, BALANCES THE DOSHAS, INCREASES THE GASTRIC FIRE, DIGESTS UNWHOLESOME FOOD AND EVEN DESTROYS DEADLY POISON.

Some of these Asanas are described as cures for different diseases. When people read this, they immediately think that Yoga Asana is a magical thing and that it can cure any kind of malady. When they come to my Ashram, they inquire, "Yogi Hari, I have this problem. Which Asana do I do for diabetes? Which Asana is for back pain?" They want an instant remedy as if they were getting a prescription. When they read things like this, they become confused and their relation to Asanas becomes superstitious. They expect miracles. But this is not based on reality. If somebody drinks poison, it is not going to do him any good if you tell him, "Go and do Mayurasana!" That would not be practical.

You can do Paschimottanasana all your life, anxiously waiting to see if Kundalini will rise. This kind of confusion abounds when people take things out of context without proper understanding.

In the system of Raja Yoga, all you need is a steady posture to sit for meditation. This does not mean any kind of steady posture. It means a steady erect posture. Otherwise people lie down on their back and they think they are meditating. If people do that, all they are doing is relaxing, lying in Savasana. Everybody can master that posture. But clearly, that is not what is meant. When you experience sitting in a steady, erect posture with your spine, neck and head in a vertical straight line, you discover that it is not so easy. You have to go through a whole series of disciplines, Asanas, proper diet, etc. It is an all encompassing process.

In that context, Hatha Yoga is used to prepare you to hold a steady, erect posture and also to help you with Pranayama because the breath eventually becomes a distraction. In fact, after you have been practicing for awhile, you will begin to observe how the breath becomes a distraction. Therefore you balance the Prana and Apana through breathing exercises and Pranayama.

Simply because you are using Hatha Yoga as a means to bring you to the state of being able to hold a steady erect posture in order to meditate, does not mean that this is the only purpose of Hatha Yoga. As you will see, the continued practice of Hatha Yoga will systematically take you to Samadhi and enlightenment.

In the same way, you can apply the spirit of Jnana Yoga to everything you do, you can also apply the spirit of Bhakti Yoga to the other systems. That is because man is a composite of all these things. You are an active person. You are an emotional, loving and feeling person. You are also an intellectual, analytical and discriminative person. So all these aspects of your personality need to be harmonized. Hence, the practice of Sampoorna Yoga. It integrates the different systems of Hatha Yoga, Jnana Yoga, Raja Yoga, Bhakti Yoga, Nada Yoga and Karma Yoga, which together harmonize the personality and greatly accelerate the purification process on all levels.

SAVASANA
Corpse Pose

34
LYING ON THE BACK LIKE A CORPSE IS CALLED SAVASANA. IT REMOVES FATIGUE AND RELAXES THE MIND.

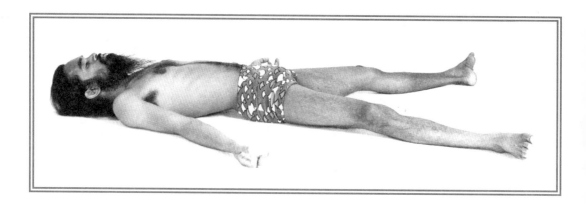

35
EIGHTY FOUR ASANAS WERE TAUGHT BY LORD SHIVA. OF THOSE, I WILL NOW DESCRIBE THE FOUR MOST IMPORTANT ONES.

Here, the Sloka states that 84 Asanas were taught. But some other sources state that there were 84,000. Others say 840,000. You just add some zeros to the 84, then you get 84,000, 840,000, and so on.

36
THESE FOUR ARE SIDDHASANA, PADMASANA, SIMHASANA AND BHADRASANA. OF THESE, SIDDHASANA IS THE BEST AND MOST COMFORTABLE.

SIDDHASANA
Adept's Pose

37
PRESS ONE HEEL AGAINST THE PERENIUM AND PLACE THE OTHER HEEL ON TOP OF THE GENITAL. SIT STEADY AND VERTICAL AND PERFORM JALANDHARA BANDHA WHILE GAZING STEADILY AT THE EYEBROW CENTER. THIS IS SIDDHASANA, WHICH FORCES OPEN THE DOOR TO LIBERATION.

Jalandhara Bandha is explained in Chapter 3, Sloka 70.

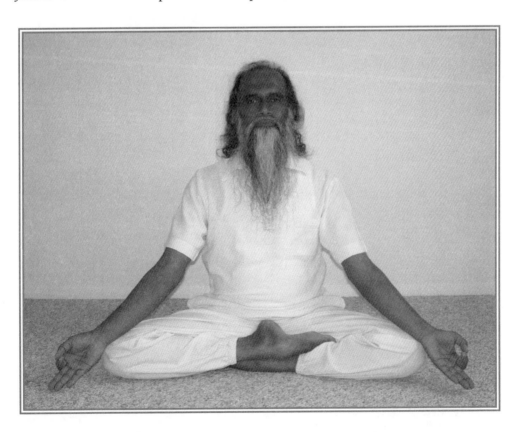

38

OTHERS PERFORM SIDDHASANA BY PLACING ONE HEEL ON THE GENITAL AND THE OTHER FOOT ON TOP OF THAT.

39

SOME REFER TO THIS ASANA AS SIDDHASANA, VAJRASANA, MUKTASANA OR GUPTASANA.

40

SIDDHASANA IS CONSIDERED TO BE FOREMOST AMONG THE ASANAS, JUST AS MODERATE DIET AND AHIMSA ARE TO THE YAMAS.

For someone to observe moderate diet is a very high stage to reach because the sense of taste is one of the hardest senses to control. Ahimsa is non-violence. In order to be non-violent, you have to be loving and kind and see the divine in all of creation. Non-violence does not only apply to people, but to all of creation, including animals, plants, etc. You cannot say that you are a non-violent person and then cut the throat of a cow, a sheep, a chicken or a goat. What kind of consciousness is that?

Siddhasana is the most important of the Asanas. It is not that the rest of the Asanas are unimportant, but you will find that in order to be able to sit in Siddhasana, you have to organize and reorganize the entire body. Remember, Gandhi used two Yamas, non-violence and truthfulness, and all the rest were subsumed in these two. It is the same with Siddhasanna.

There are other effects of Siddhasana, such as stimulating the perineum muscle and inducing Mula Bandha. In the erect posture of Siddhasana, the Prana flows very freely and nicely up the Sushumna. It also induces steadiness of mind. You will be able to sit with ease when the hips and groin are opened and the ankles and knees are flexed.

41
OUT OF THE 84 ASANAS, SIDDHASANA SHOULD ALWAYS BE PRACTICED BECAUSE IT PURIFIES THE 72,000 NADIS.

This could be very misleading if you think that just sitting in Siddhasana will purify all your Nadis. This is just a facilitator of the practices like Pranayama. In order for the Nadis to be purified, the emotions and the mind also have to be purified. It is not just a physical thing.

Some people are of the opinion that if you are able to sit in Siddhasana comfortably, your Nadis are already a little bit purified. There are people who are very flexible, such as gymnasts and acrobats, but it does not necessarily mean that their Nadis are purified. Yama and Niyama are indispensable in the process of Nadi purification.

42
THE YOGI WHO MEDITATES ON THE ATMAN, TAKES PURE AND MODERATE DIET AND PRACTICES SIDDHASANA FOR 12 YEARS, ATTAINS SIDDHI OR PERFECTION.

"Who am I?" You are the Soul, the Atman or perfection. To identify with the higher reality is to experience this perfection of who you are. This, however is a step-by-step process of refinement and purification. So to meditate on the Atman is to constantly detach the mind from the lower and attach it to the higher until all the veils are peeled off and only the Self remains. This is the state of perfection.

There is only one Yoga, one union. To reach this state, you have to go through a process. You may employ different forms of disciplines but the objective is ultimately the same: realization of the Atman, the Self or Self-Realization. This is not an exclusive goal of Jnana Yoga practice.

Similarly, meditation is not exclusive of Raja Yoga. Meditation is a state that is reached. It is not something that you do. Just like sleep is not something that you do, it is a state that you fall into. Whether you put on nice music or you sleep on a king size bed, a water bed or on the pavement, you will only fall asleep when the mind and body are relaxed. You can be on the best bed, but if the body and mind are not relaxed, you are not going to fall asleep. Similarly, you can do all kinds of Asana, but if your mind is not purified, it will not reach that state of steadiness. You will not experience your perfection.

A general misunderstanding of Hatha Yoga, Raja Yoga, Jnana Yoga, Bhakti Yoga, Nada Yoga and Karma Yoga exists. All of these systems are really only for one purpose, which is to help you refine and purify. Purification has to take place on all levels. It is not only purity of the body. There also must be purity of mind in order to bring the mind to a state of steadiness.

Considering all the purification you need to do, do you really think that 12 years to attain perfection is a long time? If you want to become a doctor, it takes 11 to 14 years. Yet people do not consider that to be too long. And what is that compared to perfection? How much discipline and Tapas must you undergo to become a doctor?

When you are involved in the discipline of Yoga, you are not experiencing hardship or discomfort. You are experiencing wonderful expansiveness of mind and consciousness. People may think, "It is so much Tapas or austerity!" But that is not the case. If you become established in moderate diet, what will you experience? You will experience good health, lightness of body and an expansive and heightened state of awareness, which is a beautiful thing.

Meditating on the Self means that you are identifying with your divine Self, your Higher Self, the Atman, which means that you are shedding all the delusions. You are becoming enlightened step-by-step. At the end of it, when you attain enlightenment or perfection, what do you get? Perfection is perfection. What more do you want than perfection? There is nothing else to attain. You are full. There is no limitation in you anymore. You have achieved everything there is to achieve.

Whereas if you study for years to become a doctor, what happens? You acquire some skills but by that time, you have grown old and tired. You are also two or three hundred thousand dollars in debt and you are completely stressed. You wonder how you are going to pay back all your loans. So you become involved in a big practice where you charge people hoards of money and you have innumerable bills and liability insurance to pay. When you initially wanted to be a doctor, you were motivated by an earnest desire to help people. Next thing you know, you are involved in all these other things, what is known as the "golden handcuffs," all of which create bondage and more negative Karma. On the other hand, the prospect of liberation should be something so enticing rather than something discouraging.

When people think of Sadhana, they become very defensive or resistant because they mistakenly think that it will be unpleasant. The prospect of giving up twelve years of your life is daunting! What will you be giving up exactly? Twelve years of indulgence, twelve years of abuse, twelve years of creating bad Karma and enslavement. But you do not think about it that way. You mistakenly look upon this as sacrifice, but in reality, it is not. On the contrary, by living a life of discipline in the spirit of Sadhana, as outlined in the Scriptures, you are actually fulfilling the higher purpose of life. You will experience fullness, whereas in the state of indulgence, you will only experience emptiness. You really have to change your vision and flip it right side up because you have been thinking upside down.

43

IF PERFECTION CAN BE ATTAINED THROUGH SIDDHASANA, THERE IS NO NEED TO PRACTICE MANY OTHER ASANAS. WHEN PRANA IS CONTROLLED, KEVALA KUMBHAKA AND UNMANI ARISE SPONTANEOUSLY.

The previous Sloka is telling you that if you meditate on the Self, you take moderate food and you practice Siddhasana for 12 years, you will reach perfection. Here it goes on to elaborate that when perfection is attainable through Siddhasana, there is no use practicing many other Asanas.

Unmani is the state of "no mind." How does that mindless state arise? First of all, the mindless state means that the mind becomes steady, calm, and there are no more ripples in the mind. What is mind? Mind is nothing but thoughts. If there is no thought, then there is no mind. Hence you reach a mindless state. That state is attained when the fluctuation of Prana ceases. Instability and fluctuation of Prana results in fluctuation of the mind. This is the relationship between Prana and the mind.

In Hatha Yoga, you strive to get control of the Prana, which naturally results in control of the mind. When that state is reached, then the breath stops spontaneously, which is called Kevala Kumbhaka and you go into the state of Unmani or "no mind." You enter a state of quietness of mind, and then you experience your oneness with the Divine. That is the ideal, the goal, the destination.

Siddhasana is the Asana that gives you stability. It also helps to awaken Kundalini Shakti and direct the energy along Sushumna for union with Shiva, Supreme Consciousness. Once the end is reached, you do not need the means anymore. All the Asanas are designed for the purpose of bringing the body into that state of ease and comfort. If you can sit steadily in Siddhasana, you can continue your other practices of Pranayama, Mudras and Bandhas in order to bring you to that state of silence. That is the process.

44

WHEN SIDDHASANA IS PERFECTED, THE THREE BANDHAS OCCUR NATURALLY AND SPONTANEOUSLY.

This is very natural when you reach that stage. For instance, when you sit straight, the energy naturally starts to flow upward. When you reach a certain level of purity and refinement in your practice, Bandhas and Mudras occur spontaneously.

Some people expect magic to happen when they practice Mudras because they have seen movies where people suddenly do miraculous things such as materializing objects and flying. I could give you all kinds of formulas, but nothing would happen if your mind is weak. On the other hand, the mind that is purified through Sadhana becomes strong. Such a mind is capable of achieving anything. It so happens that the spiritual aspirant who is guided by right discrimination, will desire liberation.

This Sloka provides some indication as to what you can expect to happen spontaneously once you have perfected Siddhasana. Bandhas are locks. In other words, they are techniques that lock in the energy and prevent the Prana generated by Pranayama from dissipating. This is the process of regulating the flow of Prana and converting it to spiritual energy. The three Bandhas are Mula Bandha, Uddiyana Bandha and Jalandhara Bandha.

45

THERE IS NO ASANA LIKE SIDDHASANA, NO KUMBHAKA LIKE KEVALA, NO MUDRA LIKE KHECHARI AND NO LAYA LIKE ANAHATA NADA.

This is a summary and statement of fact, which is clarified later on in the exposition.

P A D M A S A N A

L o t u s   P o s e

46

PLACE THE RIGHT FOOT ON THE LEFT THIGH AND THE LEFT FOOT ON THE RIGHT THIGH. CROSS THE ARMS BEHIND THE BACK AND GRAB HOLD OF THE TOES. PERFORM JALANDHARA BANDHA AND GAZE AT THE TIP OF THE NOSE. THIS IS PADMASANA AND IT DESTROYS ALL OF THE YOGI'S DISEASES.

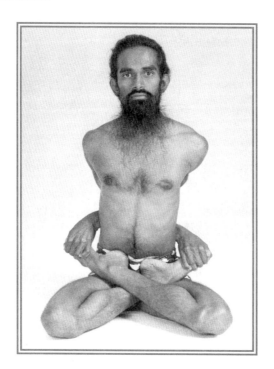

47

PLACE THE FEET ON THE THIGHS WITH THE SOLES UPWARDS AND PLACE THE HANDS ON THE SOLES WITH THE PALMS UPWARDS.

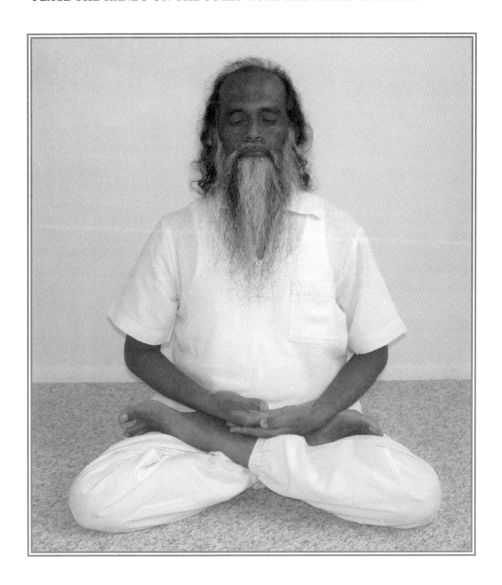

48

**GAZE AT THE TIP OF THE NOSE KEEPING THE TONGUE PRESSED
AGAINST THE ROOT OF THE UPPER TEETH. APPLY JALANDHARA BAND-
HA AND SLOWLY RAISE THE PRANA UPWARDS.**

49

**THIS PADMASANA DESTROYS ALL DISEASES. ORDINARY PEOPLE CAN-
NOT ACHIEVE IT. ONLY A FEW WISE ONES ON EARTH CAN.**

There are so many acrobats and gymnasts who can do perfect Padmasana in all its
variations, but does that mean that they are the few wise people on earth? This is
to encourage you to do your practice so that you are able to sit in Padmasana.

50

**SIT IN PADMASANA WITH THE ONE PALM IN THE OTHER AND CONCEN-
TRATE ON THE SELF. WITH EVERY INHALATION, APPLY JALANDHARA
AND MULA BANDHA TO DRAW THE APANA UP AND PRESS THE PRANA
DOWN. BY JOINING THE PRANA AND APANA AT THE NAVEL, THE SHAK-
TI IS AWAKENED AND ONE GETS THE HIGHEST KNOWLEDGE.**

While sitting in Padmasana, you mentally draw the Apana up with Mula Bandha
and send the Prana down with Jalandhara Bandha, and then there will be compres-
sion and explosion. This will not come spontaneously. You have to practice this.

51
**THE YOGI WHO CONTROLS THE BREATH WHILE SITTING IN PAD-
MASANA IS FREE FROM BONDAGE WITHOUT A DOUBT.**

Simhasana
Lion Pose

52
**PLACE THE ANKLES BELOW THE GENITAL WITH THE RIGHT ANKLE ON
THE RIGHT SIDE AND THE LEFT ANKLE ON THE LEFT SIDE OF THE
PERENIUM.**

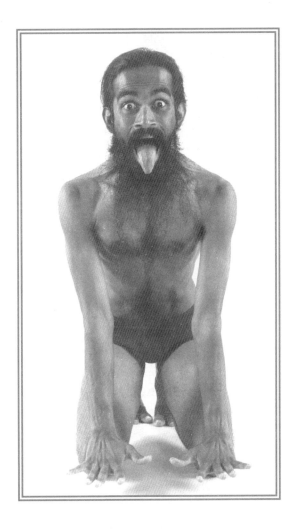

53

**PRESS THE PALMS ON THE KNEES WITH THE FINGERS SPREAD APART.
EXHALE FORCEFULLY WITH THE MOUTH WIDE OPEN AND WHILE
HOLDING THE BREATH EXTERNALLY, GAZE ON THE THIRD EYE WITH A
CONCENTRATED MIND.**

54

**THIS IS SIMHASANA AND IS HELD IN HIGH ESTEEM BY GREAT YOGIS.
THIS EXCELLENT ASANA FACILITATES THE THREE BANDHAS.**

Simhasana should be performed by extending the tongue out as far as you can, opening the eyes wide and roaring like a lion on the exhale. In this posture, the Bandhas are naturally induced. It also helps to reverse the introverted nature of shy people and loosen inhibitions. As you can see, these nuances of the postures are not included in the Sloka. That is why it is so important to have the instruction of a knowledgeable Guru to guide you. In this way, you will get the maximum benefit from the posture.

BHADRASANA

Gracious Pose

55-56

IN A SITTING POSITION, BRING THE SOLES OF THE FEET TOGETHER. INTERLACE THE FINGERS AND CUP THE TOES. PULL THE HEELS TO THE GROIN. PUSH THE CHEST FORWARD, HEAD AND ELBOWS BACK AND BREATHE DEEPLY. THIS IS BHADRASANA WHICH DESTROYS ALL DISEASES. THE SIDDHAS CALL IT GORAKSHASANA.

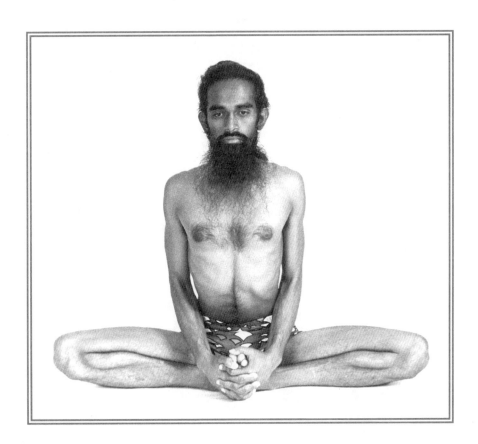

57

HAVING PASSED THE STAGE OF FATIGUE IN THE PRACTICE OF ASANAS AND BANDHAS, THE YOGI SHOULD PRACTICE PURIFICATION OF THE NADIS, MUDRAS AND PRANAYAMA.

58

THE SEQUENCE OF HATHA YOGA IS, PRACTICE OF ASANAS, THE VARIOUS KUMBHAKAS, MUDRAS AND CONCENTRATION ON THE ANAHATA NADA.

Through the various Asanas, Kumbhakas (which are the retention of breath in breathing exercises), Mudras and Bandhas, all the systems and Nadis are purified and refined, and then your mind becomes indrawn, withdrawn and concentrated. Then you are able to experience the Anahata sound, which will further take the mind to that state of transcendence. That is the sequence.

YOGIC DIET

59

A BRAHMACHARI WHO TAKES MODERATE AND PURE FOOD, IS INTENT AND CONSISTENT IN HIS PRACTICE OF YOGA AND RENUNCIATION, BECOMES A SIDDHA AFTER A YEAR WITHOUT A DOUBT.

This is a clear outline of the stages of perfection and how the process is accelerated. In Sloka 42, it states that, "The Yogi who meditates on the Atman, takes pure and moderate diet and practices Siddhasana for 12 years, attains perfection." In this Sloka, the Yogi is referred to as Brahmachari, one whose study and practice is solely devoted to self-knowledge, who has complete control of the senses, is established in the sublimation of the sexual energy, is consistent and steady in his practice, and is firm in renunciation. Such a Yogi, a Brahmachari, becomes a Siddha in one year. This is understandable considering this person has fulfilled all his obligations, his mind is completely turned away from the world, he is living in seclusion, and he is involved in practice according to the Scriptures and instructions of his Guru. It means that his mind is not distracted but constantly meditating and identifying with the Atman.

60
MODERATE DIET MEANS AGREEABLE AND SWEET FOOD THAT IS TAKEN AS AN OFFERING TO GOD WITH A QUARTER OF THE STOMACH EMPTY.

Master Sivananda said you should be a little hungry all the time. The stomach must not be overloaded. Most people are like infants when it comes to eating. They continue to eat until they are so full that the food starts coming back up. They also suffer from constipation and other disgestive problems. The solution is to take agreeable food in moderation.

The Sloka says that sweet food should be taken "as an offering to God." Most people consume food without giving it a second thought. Others will take their time in growing it or purchasing it from a supermarket, preparing it and even savoring it. Food plays such an important role in our lives but do we really understand what food is and its purpose, other than the fact that we enjoy eating it and need it to stay alive? How conscious are we about the food we eat?

The *Taittiriya Upanishad* tells us about the divine origin of food:

> *"From that which is the Atman came space; from space, air; from air, fire; from fire, water; from water, earth; from earth, plants; from plants, food; and from food the human body with all the organs of action and perception. All beings are made of food, which becomes food again for other beings after death. From that standpoint, food is therefore the best medicine for all the body's ailments. From food are made all bodies. All bodies feed on food, which becomes food for other beings after death. Those who meditate on food as Brahman will never lack life's comforts.*
>
> *Human beings, beast and bird live by breath. Breath is therefore the true sign of life. It is the life force that is called Prana in everyone. That determines how long we are to live. Those who would look upon Prana as the Lord's gift shall live to complete the full span of life."*

So what does this mean? Food comes from the Divine source. It is part of an evolution of consciousness, although some prefer to think about it in terms of devolution, from the One Supreme Consciousness known as Brahman to subsequent levels. Space was created through the big bang from one unit, the ultimate source. Subsequently, as space expanded, consciousness moved level by level, until eventually "food" manifested. Food is the substance of which the physical body is composed. That is why the physical body is called the food sheath in Vedanta philosophy. This food sheath or Annamaya Kosha, in turn, becomes food for other living organisms. It is a continuous ongoing process that happens even while we are alive. Innumerable germs and bacteria are constantly feeding on and processing us. We co-exist in a symbiotic relationship. If we kill all the bacteria within us, we would die.

The moment we die, decomposition starts, which is simply bacteria, germs and worms eating and processing us. The physical body is recycled and becomes food again, even before it enters the earth. The *Taittiriya Upanishad* goes on further to state, "From food are born all creatures, by food they grow, and to food they return." The physical body came from food and it returns to food. It is simply not true that we are only ashes and dust! Others sustain us and we sustain others. All of these beings come from the same divine source. It is a continuous chain of consciousness. When you eat, you are consuming the Divine. Everything is consciousness, no matter what level it is. When you eat, you are ingesting the consciousness of the food and it will become part of you. The energy consciousness in your body will also nourish the divine organisms that feed off of you. One needs to meditate on the mystical nature of food to fully grasp and appreciate it.

The *Taittiriya Upanishad* goes on further to talk about the connection between food and Prana. The body returns to the elements when the Prana or life force leaves it. Death of the physical body is like shedding clothes. The soul, the Self, never dies. Therefore we still exist beyond the physical form after we die. But while we are alive, we need food and Prana to sustain us.

Prana is part of the vital sheath, or energy sheath, which is present within the physical body. There is an immediate relationship between food and Prana. The quality of the Prana depends on the kind of food we eat. That, in turn, determines the condition of the mind, which is a Yogi's main field of action. A Yogi therefore works on all three bodies: the physical body, which is composed of the food sheath; the astral body, which is composed of the energy, mental and intellectual sheaths; and the causal body, which is composed of the blissful sheath. All five sheaths are interrelated and affect one another.

The soul in the human embodiment is conditioned by the physical body, senses, emotions, mind, intellect, ego and the causal body. We are the Self, the experiencer or the passenger, riding in the chariot or the physical body. A nice imagery is used in the *Bhagavad Gita* to illustrate this. The chariot is the physical body, the horses are the senses, the reins are the mind, the charioteer is the intellect, and the soul is the passenger going wherever the mind and senses lead it. If the intellect is not keen and discriminating, it will not know where to guide the chariot and its passenger. In that case, the mind will not be able to hold the reins. The horses or the senses will take over and rage out of control. That is when the passenger or the Self is placed in jeopardy. Even the chariot or the physical body will be jeopardized and at risk of breaking.

The *Upanishad* points out that the physical body is a gift of God and should be cared for accordingly. Only then shall we "never lack life's comforts" necessary to do Sadhana. The physical body is the food sheath. So it is clear that food is very important and we should relate to food as divine.

Therefore, preliminary in every spiritual discipline is caring for the body. Without good health, it will be difficult to focus on spiritual practices. Sickness or "disease" will agitate the mind, a condition you want to avoid since Yoga is the process of gaining perfect control of the mind.

Knowledge of food and diet is the first priority for a Yogic practitioner. There is no need to become obsessed about diet but a number of general rules and guidelines must be respected in order to experience good health.

Diet should be adapted to one's constitution. Different people have different constitutions and need different kinds of food. Ayurveda, the traditional medicine in India, distinguishes three major qualities by which people's constitutions are determined: Vata, Pitta and Kapha or a combination thereof. Food that is agreeable to a person of a Vata constitution is not necessarily agreeable to someone of a Pitta constitution. It might even be harmful. A basic knowledge of one's constitution helps to avert problems and correct certain conditions.

There is another kind of constitution known as the Manas Prakriti, which is of the utmost importance to the Yogi. These are Sattwa, Rajas and Tamas. A spiritual aspirant tries to refine and purify his personality in order to move away from grossness and become more subtle. As food also has an effect on the mind, he will therefore have to pay attention to what he eats. The more refined and purified one becomes, the more immediate the effect of wrong diet. That is why on a more advanced level, one is dealing with subtle vibrations. At that stage, one can even feel the vibrations of the conciousness of the cook in the food at the time he cooks. People who cook in restaurants are often stressed and may even be exploited by greedy owners. The corruption thus created in their minds is transmitted to the food in the form of bad vibrations. This process is similar to the descentof the Supreme Consciousness, Brahman, and its final manifestation as food, which makes up the body. If the consciousness of the people preparing the food is contaminated, the one eating it will consume that bad energy. That is why when you are preparing food, you should prepare it with love and offer blessings before you eat it.

It is important to study the qualities of food. The *Bhagavad Gita* directs us on the way:

> *"The food which is agreeable to different people is of three sorts. Sattwic people like foods that increase their prana, energy, strength, purity, joy and health. Such foods add to the pleasure and cheerfulness of physical and mental life. They are juicy, soothing, fresh and agreeable. Rajasic people prefer foods that are bitter, sour, salty, hot, pungent, acid and burning. These cause ill health, pain, grief and misery. Tamasic people take pleasure in foods that are stale, tasteless, putrid and impure. They like to eat the leftovers of others."*

Whereas the principles of Ayurveda refer to the constitution of the body, the Manas Prakriti refers to the constitution and the state of the mind. Here also, three qualities are distinguished: Tamas, Rajas and Sattwa. They are referred to as the three Gunas. These three principles are present in everything, including nature, the mind and food.

Tamas refers to laziness, inertia and darkness. In nature, Tamas is all that is heavy and solid, like rocks. People of a Tamasic nature are gross, lazy and dull. Food that is stale, overripe, reheated or that induces dullness are Tamasic. Examples are meat and alcohol. They make one dull and lazy and induce negative thoughts.

Rajas refers to activity and dynamics. In nature, it manifests as storm, thunder and lightning. Rajasic people are restless, motivated by greed and pursue success and power. In food, it refers to everything that is too spicy, bitter or sour. Examples are spices, coffee, tea, onions and garlic. They agitate the mind, making it difficult for the Yogi to meditate or to maintain a focused, peaceful mind.

Sattwa is purity. In nature, it represents everything that is beautiful and peaceful. Sattwic people are peaceful, calm, focused and pure in heart and mind. Sattwic food is healthy food, such as fresh fruits and vegetables, grains, whole bread, whole rice, milk, ghee, sprouts, honey and herbal tea. A Sattwic diet is most beneficial to a Yogic practitioner because it helps to develop Sattwa in his personality.

Pure diet is very important in the practice of Hatha Yoga because a Yogi exists on a very subtle balance. His objective is to gain control of the mind. This is attained through the purification of body, senses and mind. As the Nadis become purified, one starts to feel the subtle vibrations of the Prana in the body. These help to still and focus the mind until one reaches the ultimate goal of transcendence and experience of the true Self.

Exotic food does not serve the spiritual aspirant. He needs simple food. Otherwise his entire practice will be consumed with correcting the imbalances that were created from ingesting such food. The spiritual aspirant should bypass Tamasic and Rajasic food and eat only Sattwic food. Eating properly, at the right time, in the right way and cultivating right habits are all ways to accelerate the purification process and spiritual evolution. Along with practicing Asanas, Pranayama and right thinking, a pure diet substantially hastens this process. Without proper knowledge and understanding, people have the tendency to eat according to their desires and habits. This practice should be abandoned. Instead, one should turn to Sattwic food. After all, one should eat pure foods "as an offering to God." For the spiritual aspirant, the body is the temple of God and to eat non-vegetarian and junk food would be a desecration of this temple. He wants to keep this temple as clean and pure as possible.

FOODS INJURIOUS TO A YOGI

61

THE FOODS THAT ARE CONSIDERED UNSUITABLE FOR A YOGI ARE BIT-TER, SOUR, PUNGENT, SALTY, HEATING, GREEN VEGETABLES THAT ARE HARD TO DIGEST, SOUR GRUEL, OIL, SESAME, MUSTARD, ALCOHOL, FISH, MEAT, CURDS, BUTTERMILK, HORSE GRAM, FRUIT OF JUJUBE, OIL CAKE, ASAFETIDA AND GARLIC.

This section informs you about food and things that will be disagreeable to you. These instructions are meant for that special time in your life when you can devote all your time to Sadhana. You are no longer living with others and you are not involved in the world, Rajasic work, etc. Therefore, this Sloka is not to be taken out of that context. You may wonder why the food described here is prohibited. It is because it is Rajasic and Tamasic in nature and will create impurities and agitate the body and mind.

62

FOOD THAT HAS BEEN REHEATED, STALE, DRY, EXCESSIVELY SALTY, ACIDIC AND A MIXTURE OF TOO MANY VEGETABLES SHOULD BE AVOIDED.

Food that is reheated and stale is tamasic and depleted of Prana. Dry, salty, acidic foods aggravate Vata and Pitta (two of the Tridoshas in Ayurveda), and therefore

disturb the metabolism. For example, dry fruits, apples, melons, potatoes, tomatoes, eggplant, ice cream, peas and green salad aggravate Vata and should be avoided by someone with a Vata imbalance. Spicy foods, peanut butter, sour fruits,
bananas, papyayas and tomatoes aggravate Pitta and should be avoided by someone with a Pitta constitution.

As a general rule, you should not mix too many vegetables or fruits together. In
fruit salad, for example, people tend to mix in a variety of fruits. But certain melons should never be combined with other fruits because they will clog the intestines and prevent proper absorption. In general, acidic fruits should never be
mixed with sweet fruits because the combination causes gas, bloating and discomfort. A simple rule to remember about melon, for instance, is to "eat it alone or
leave it alone." Another important principle is to eat seasonal food that is grown
locally, which is also advised if you are following a macrobiotic diet. The intelligence of nature is indisputable. It is divine consciousness, providing everything at
the right time and in the right locality. Melons do not grow in winter. They grow
in summer because we are supposed to eat them when we feel hot and thirsty.

The very same food can have three phases. A fruit that is ripening, still green, sour
and pungent is of a Rajisic nature. When it is ripe and ready to pluck from the
tree, it is Sattwic. At that point, one must hardly pull the fruit from the tree; it
harvests itself. When a fruit is overripe, it turns Tamasic. If you eat a mango at the
opportune time, you can actually feel the Prana in the body. The moment you put
a ripe mango in your mouth, instantly the senses wake up and the Prana explodes
in your body and mind. Sattwic food is juicy, sweet and agreeable.

Without thinking, you eat everything that is put on the table like a vacuum cleaner. But that creates all kinds of problems. You should therefore adhere to these simple rules in order to purify your bodily systems and keep the mind from becoming agitated.

63
GORAKSHANATH ADVISED TO AVOID BAD COMPANY, MIXING WITH THE OPPOSITE SEX, BATHING EARLY IN THE MORNING, FASTING, LONG PILGRIMAGES, SITTING IN FRONT OF THE FIRE AND OVER EXERTION.

These are the things that should be avoided so that you do not deplete the Prana or agitate the mind. Avoiding "bad company" essentially means disassociating from people who are not on the same spiritual path like yourself because it may deplete your energy and degrade your consciousness.

Mixing with the opposite sex will excite the mind and pull the energy to the lower Chakras.

The instruction to avoid "bathing in the morning" stems from the fact that they did not have running hot water in those days. When you take a cold shower in the morning, it shocks the psychic and Pranic Systems, and then you cannot meditate.

Long pilgrimages, fasting and exertion will make you tired. You need the energy for Sadhana. When you reach the point in your Sadhana when you are practicing intensely, you increase the gastric fire, and therefore fasting will create problems.

You should avoid fire because it drains your energy. People like to sit in front of camp fires and by their fire places. Then they wonder why they feel so tired afterward.

Foods Most Beneficial to a Yogi

64
THE MOST BENEFICIAL FOOD FOR THE YOGI ARE GOOD GRAINS, WHEAT, RICE, BARLEY, MILK, GHEE, BROWN RICE, SUGAR CANDY, HONEY, DRIED GINGER, PATOLA FRUIT, FIVE VEGETABLES, MUNG AND SIMILAR PULSES AND PURE WATER.

These foods will promote Sattwa, give energy and not excite the mind. In order to prepare a Sattwic meal, one also has to have proper knowledge about how to cook. Sattwic vegetables that are overcooked, for instance, become Tamasic and drained of all the Prana. A Yogi will feel it as poison in his body.

A general guideline is to eat organic food that is grown with love and respect for nature. One should stay away from canned, processed and frozen food as much as possible because Prana is lost when food is treated this way. By radiating food, all the bacteria are killed in order to preserve the food longer. This, however, has nothing to do with enhancing nutrition. It is done for commercial reasons only.

65
A YOGI SHOULD TAKE SWEET AND PLEASING FOOD MIXED WITH GHEE AND MILK. IT SHOULD BE SUITABLE AND NOURISHING TO THE DHATUS.

What constitutes "sweet and pleasing food" is a subject of debate and may depend on the individual's constitution and sensitivity to certain foods. Of course in the West, there are several schools of thoughts. People are vegetarian, lacto vegetarian, vegan, etc. The food a Yogi consumes should nourish the Dhatus, which are the seven vital tissues that work together to ensure a good functioning of the body. Your diet should consist of Sattwic food, which will naturally nourish the Dhatus.

It is a big misunderstanding that healthy, vegetarian food is tasteless. The *Bhagavad Gita* clearly states that Sattwic food is "juicy, soothing, fresh and agreeable." That is why we have the senses at our disposal. They serve to tell us which foods are healthy and which foods we should avoid. The sense of smell informs us whether food is rotten or stale so that we become aware that it is bad for the body and discard it. Taste tells us whether food is saturated with Prana or whether it is corrupted. Our sight equally helps to distinguish whether food is agreeable or disagreeable. That is what the senses are designed for and that is why they need protection. If you understand that the senses are an extension of the mind, you will try to discipline and protect them. When the nose is constantly used to smell perfume, the sense of smell becomes blunted and deranged. It will not serve its original purpose of helping to distinguish between healthy and unhealthy food anymore.

The excessive use of vitamins and supplements is another kind of derangement. Healthy, organic, Sattwic food that is not corrupted by pesticides contains all the vitamins and nourishment a body needs.

Some people tell you not to take milk because milk is very bad for you. But milk is good for you if you are involved in this kind of Sadhana. Jesus taught that the milk of animals is given by God to man as food but that their flesh is not. He strictly and emphatically forbid eating meat but recommended drinking milk. Ghee is recommended here because it is very good for detoxification.

66
ANYONE CAN ATTAIN PERFECTION THROUGH THE DILIGENT AND SYS-
TEMATIC PRACTICE OF YOGA REGARDLESS OF WHETHER HE IS YOUNG,
OLD, VERY OLD, SICK OR FEEBLE.

Therefore anybody can do Yoga!

67
SUCCESS IN YOGA IS ATTAINED ONLY THROUGH PRACTICE AND NOT
BY MERELY READING BOOKS.

People who are just reading and translating Yogic texts without any experience will create problems. It generates confusion in the minds of peolpe because they expound on things without indepth experience of the subject matter.

Practice what your Guru teaches you. Master Sivananda says, "An ounce of practice is worth more than tons of theory." Notice that he does not say that it is worth tons of theory but "more than" tons of theory. Only information or teaching that is put into practice is worth anything.

68

PERFECTION IS NOT ATTAINED BY MERELY TALKING ABOUT IT OR WEARING A PARTICULAR GARB OR ATTIRE. ONLY THROUGH PRACTICE WILL ONE ATTAIN PERFECTION. THIS IS THE TRUTH WITHOUT A DOUBT.

Just because you put on a robe or special attire does not make you a Yogi per se.

69

ASANA, PRANAYAMA, BANDHAS, MUDRAS AND ALL THE VARIOUS DISCIPLINES IN HATHA YOGA MUST BE PRACTICED UNTIL THE HIGHEST STATE OF PERFECTION THAT IS CALLED RAJA YOGA IS ATTAINED.

It is taken for granted that you are already established in Yama and Niyama. As a human being who has reached the state where you practice Yoga with this intensity and dedication, there should not be any battle, struggle, fight or problems with Yama and Niyama. If you are living alone practicing Yoga when you still have all kinds of greed, hatred, lust, jealousy, envy and fear, it means that you need therapy and that you should go to a psychiatrist instead of retreating into a hermitage to do Yoga. It means that you are not yet fit to live alone to practice Yoga. Those lower emotions must be eradicated in order to be able to have that kind of committment.

Chapter Two

PRANAYAMA

1

**AFTER GAINING CONTROL OF BODY AND SENSES THROUGH THE PRAC-
TICE OF ASANA AND OBSERVING A PURE AND MODERATE DIET, THE
YOGI SHOULD PRACTICE PRANAYAMA ACCORDING TO THE INSTRUC-
TIONS OF THE GURU.**

A cursory reading of this Sloka may leave the wrong impression that breathing
exercises should be practiced only after one has mastered the Asanas. In fact, this
is a common misunderstanding in certain schools of Yoga that do not teach
breathing exercises until the students have practiced Asanas for years. But this is a
gross blunder in the practice of Hatha Yoga. While it is true that Pranayama,
which means the control of Prana, can only be practiced after you have reached a
very high level in your Sadhana in terms of refinement and purity of the Nadis, it
does not mean that you should not practice breathing exercises.

Analysis of the breathing process compels one to practice breathing exercises from
the very inception. Breathing occurs through the contraction and expansion of
muscles, such as the diaphragm, abdominals, chest and intercostal muscles, which
are all involved in the practice of Asanas. The quality of breathing depends on
one's ability to expand and contract these muscles. The more one is able to expand
them, the more space is created in the lungs, the easier it is to inhale and the more
fresh air and oxygen is taken in for circulation to the blood and nourishment of
the body's tissues. The more one can contract these muscles, the more air will be
expelled. It is impossible to squeeze out all the air in the lungs because you cannot collapse the lungs. With the development of these respiratory muscles, the
residual stale air that remains will diminish significantly.

In recent times, people have lost contact with their breath and the diaphragm has become a neglected muscle. But fortunately in the practice of Yoga, the diaphragm is exercised just like any other muscle. Most of us do not use our breathing capacities efficiently to exchange stale air for fresh air in the lungs. As a result, toxins accumulate in the body, causing ailments such as headaches, exhaustion and laziness. Once this is understood, one can easily see the need to practice breathing exercises from the very onset of Asana practice.

Regular practice leads to enhanced concentration and increased focused attention, which are attributes that can then be applied to every day life.

That is why, in Sampoorna Yoga, you are involved in an integrated practice. Through breathing exercises, the Prana or life-force is enhanced. Warming up exercises tone the body and create strength and endurance. This is followed by a systematic practice of Yoga postures or Asanas, which work on all the systems of the body. This systematic approach to Hatha Yoga develops the individual in a harmonious and balanced way. *(See "Hatha Yoga" in "Sampoorna Yoga," a book by Yogi Hari.)* On the other hand, performing only one or two Asanas over an extended period of time creates imbalance in the body.

Breathing exercises are an integral part of a systematic approach and are performed from the time one starts with Yoga Asanas. Set forth below are the techniques for breathing exercises and Pranayama. In each case, you should breathe through the nose because receptors of Prana are also in the upper part of the nose.

Abdominal Breathing:

You should commence your practice with abdominal breath to learn how to use the diaphragm. This practice also improves attention and concentration.

Technique: Sit comfortably with your spine, neck and head in a vertical straight line. Place one hand on your belly to develop awareness and focus. Start with a complete exhalation by contracting the abdominal muscles and the diaphragm. Then inhale slowly, pushing the abdomen out while the rest of the body is relaxed. Make sure you do not use the chest to breathe. Exhale completely by slowly contracting your abdomen towards the spine. Make your exhalation twice as long as your inhalation. Continue this for a few minutes.

One should try to develop the habit of always breathing abdominally. The abdominal breath helps to reduce stress. The average person breathes heavily in the chest in times of stress. By consciously breathing abdominally, you will notice a considerable calming effect on your body, mind and emotions. Once you master the abdominal breath, you can move on to abdominal and chest breathing.

Abdominal and Chest Breathing:

Here you can combine abdominal breathing with chest breathing.

Technique: Sit comfortably with your spine, neck and head in a vertical straight line. Breathe abdominally as described above, but this time keep that air in the abdomen and continue to breathe into the chest by expanding the rib cage. In the exhalation, start relaxing the chest only and then subsequently squeeze out all the air from the abdomen. Do this practice for a few minutes. Once this becomes comfortable you can proceed to Full Yogic Breathing.

Full Yogic Breath:

Full Yogic Breath combines abdominal and chest breathing with a further expansion of the lungs.

Technique: Follow the first two stages as described above and then proceed to inhale deeper while further expanding the chest and lifting the shoulders slightly. You exhale in the reverse order, by lowering the shoulders first, followed by relaxing the chest and finally squeezing all the air out from your belly. Once you have reached this stage in your practice, you can do the Full Yogic Breath for 3 to 5 minutes every sitting.

The Full Yogic Breath is very energizing and can be practiced at any time and anywhere, provided that the air is not polluted and you do not practice after eating.

Kapalabati:

Kapalabhati is a cleansing breath. Even though it is considered to be one of the Kriyas or cleansing practices that will be discussed later on in this book, Kapalabhati is included as a breathing exercise in the Sampoorna Hatha Yoga practice from the very onset because it strengthens the muscles of the diaphram, abdomen and chest. The cleansing effect arises from the forceful exhalation, which removes more stale air from the lungs. The lungs are very important for the elimination of toxins. Kapalabhati also helps people to extinguish bad habits such as smoking.

Technique: Sit comfortably with your back, neck and head in a vertical straight line. Inhale deeply and exhale forcefully through the nose 30 times, the way you would blow your nose. The air will rush in automatically, therefore there is no need to inhale consciously between exhalations. Prolong the last exhalation. Then energize the body by inhaling deeply while pushing the arms out to the sides and expanding the chest. Let your head hang backwards and rotate the wrists. Exhale slowly while bringing the palms together. Fill up the lungs comfortably and retain the breath for 30 counts. Close your eyes and focus your attention on the point between the eyebrows, the third eye, the Ajna Chakra. Exhale slowly and completely. Take a Full Yogic Breath. This is one round of Kapalabhati. Practice three rounds. Once this becomes comfortable, gradually increase the number of exhalations and retentions.

The quality of breathing is closely connected with the focus of mind while practicing Asanas. If you can consciously manipulate the respiratory muscles, you will be able to affect breathing and gain control over your breath. You do not have to wait until you reach perfection in Asana practice and the body becomes completely refined and free from tension and stress to start breathing exercises.

By following this systematic approach, when a Yogi reaches an advanced level in his Asana practice, he is already practicing breathing exercises. These are not considered as Pranayama because that term refers to the actual control of Prana, the life-force. But control of Prana does not happen suddenly. You cannot simply turn on a switch after having practiced Asanas for years and expect to control the Prana. Having gained control of the breathing mechanisms, one can proceed to more evolved practices of Pranayama.

Sampoorna Yoga will take you step-by-step in your Sadhana and evolution.

A Yogi should also take moderate and Sattwic diet. As you continue your practice of Asana and Pranayama and become aware of what proper health is, naturally you will feel the effect of food on your well-being and it will become an integral part of your discipline.

2
WHEN THE BREATHING IS DISTURBED, THE MIND IS DISTURBED.
WHEN THE BREATH IS CONTROLLED, THE MIND IS UNDER CONTROL.
THUS, ONE SHOULD GAIN CONTROL OF THE BREATH.

Again in this new chapter, as with any sacred Scripture, the objective is explained in the very beginning. If you do not have a clear understanding about why you are doing something, then you will practice blindly.

As Maharishi Patanjali states in one of his first Sutras, "Yoga Chitta Vritti Nirodha." Yoga is the control of all thought waves in the mind. That is the goal, the ideal as defined in *The Yoga Sutras of Patanjali.* Every form of Sadhana and discipline should serve to reduce agitation in the mind. That state of the highest union is reached when the mind becomes steady and still and when there is no more movement of Chitta (the mind).

Regardless of what discipline one is involved in, Yoga should contribute to control of the mind through acquiring focus and concentration. This is an important process in Hatha Yoga.

In the Hatha Yoga approach, the mind is controlled by gaining control over the vital energy or Prana through control of the breath. Proper breathing brings more oxygen to the blood and thus to the brain, and helps one to gain control of the Prana. The goal remains the same as in other Yoga paths, but in this system, it is reached through the control of Prana because of the close relationship between mind and Prana. The Prana is the flywheel of the mind. When the Prana is disturbed, the mind becomes disturbed and more restless. In the same way, when the mind is disturbed, breathing becomes labored, agitated and shallow. When the breath is calm, the mind is also steady.

3

AS LONG AS THERE IS BREATH IN THE BODY, THERE IS LIFE. DEATH IS WHEN THE BREATH STOPS. THEREFORE, ONE SHOULD GAIN CONTROL OF THIS BREATH.

Prana is more than air and oxygen. It is the life-force. It is the subtle vital energy that is ever present and can be found everywhere. It is the same in a tree, an animal or a human being. Prana flows through the Nadis into the mind and body and nourishes the bodily systems, thereby keeping us alive and animated. We do not know what it is and we have never seen it, but when somebody dies, we say that the life has left the body.

The Yogi strives to maintain and increase the flow of Prana in the body. When the amount of Prana in the body is increased and enhanced, the person is vibrant and alive. But when the Prana is attenuated or weak, the person appears lifeless or near death. It is believed that each being has a fixed amount of breath in his lifetime, and once it is used up, that being dies. Thus the Yogi, through gaining control of the breath, is able to prolong life.

In the human body, the Prana is harnessed through a very intricate and important breathing mechanism. Prana can be accessed everywhere through this breathing mechanism. Air enters the body through the nose and travels through the larynx, trachea, bronchi, bronchioles and alveoli, where an exchange of oxygen and carbon dioxide takes place between the lungs and the blood. The heart pumps blood containing carbon dioxide, gas and waste to the lungs for expulsion and receives Prana and oxygen that is then circulated to the body. The diaphragm, abdominals, intercostals and chest muscles are sed in breathing, which enable the body to inhale more fresh air and oxygen and to expel stale air.

Since Prana is also absorbed through the nose, it affects us when we smell something horrible. The perfume and deodorants people use are actually very toxic for the system. People are poisoning themselves without being aware of it. After awhile, the sense of smell is turned off. This intricate and sensitive mechanism that God has given us must be respected and protected.

The life-force or Prana has different names according to its function in the body. Every upward or inward movement of energy is called Prana. Every downward or outward movement, as in the excretion of waste, is called Apana. Udana removes the life-force at death. Samana is the energy functioning in the middle region of the body and digests the food. Vyana is the force that distributes the nutrients throughout the body through circulation.

A Yogi who understands these principles knows which form of Prana is out of balance by observing the symptoms of imbalance. He can then regulate his lifestyle and Sadhana accordingly and take foods and herbs that either increase or lower the specific Prana to restore balance.

For instance, when you cannot go to the bathroom, Apana is not functioning properly. Having to go too often or developing hemorrhoids is indicative of an excess of Apana. In case of digestive problems, Samana is out of balance. Through this kind of awareness, a Yogi can regulate his diet and practice to maintain a balance, thus maintaining good health.

4

IF THE PRANA DOES NOT FLOW THROUGH THE SUSHUMNA BECAUSE OF IMPURITIES OF THE NADIS, HOW CAN UNMANI ARISE AND HOW CAN THE GOAL BE REACHED?

Here, the Scripture emphasizes a major obstacle to liberation, namely the impurities in the Nadis. When the Nadis are purified through Hatha Yoga, then the Prana can gain free passage through the most important Nadi, the Sushumna, which is in the central passage in the Chakra system. Yogic exercises, Pranayama and a purified mind cause the Prana to flow unblocked through the Sushumna Nadi. When this happens, the Kundalini Shakti, lying dormant at the root or Muladhara Chakra, is awakened. Once the Sushumna is purified, Kundalini Shakti can rise up to the Sahasrara Chakra, the highest Chakra at the crown of the head, where the individual consciousness merges with the Supreme Consciousness. At that point, one identifies with the Higher Self, the true Self. That is when the state of Yoga is reached. One experiences the ocean of consciousness that underlies the whole of existence and which is the true reality. This is a mindless state, a state of pure experience.

"Unmani," or that state of "no mind" will not arise unless the Prana is controlled. There will be fluctuation of thoughts until one reaches the state where the Prana flows through the Sushumna in the central passage of the energy system, which functions in the physical body as the spinal chord.

The Pingala and Ida Nadis are located on either side of the Sushumna and relate to the sympathetic and parasympathetic ganglia in the spinal column. While the Prana is flowing through the Pingala and Ida Nadis, the positive and negative poles, or the sun and the moon, one will experience the state of duality, characterized by mental fluctuation. When the Prana flows through Sushumna, one experiences a state of peacefulness and quietness of mind.

This will not happen unless the Nadis are purified. Sadhana is the way to purify the Nadis. This does not involve just doing Asanas or eating good food. A proper practice is an integrated one, founded on observing the Yamas and Niyamas, as was explained in the previous chapter.

5

THE YOGI EXPERIENCES THE FLOW OF PRANA WHEN THE NADIS ARE PURIFIED.

Pranayama refers to the ability to control Prana and direct that energy consciously. Energy is needed to maintain the functions of body and mind. But until one gains control over the Prana, it will just be flowing in and out. The Prana must be replenished continuously. That is why the more impurities there are in the body and mind, the faster people breathe. When the mind and body are purified, the breath subsides because there is less need to breathe. One can sit quietly and comfortably. At this stage, one can actually feel the flow of Prana through the body. One can harness that Prana, store it, use it when needed and direct it wherever needed.

When Asanas are practiced for the first time, the breathing is heavy. As the Nadis are purified and the body becomes more refined, the breathing becomes very rhythmic and slow. Even in headstand, one will eventually be able to breathe only two or three times a minute and very calmly.

The same process takes place in meditation. In the beginning, the effort to concentrate is distracted by the breath. After awhile, it becomes very soft and slow and eventually reaches a point when, in the state of Samadhi, the breath is suspended.

Perfection does not come suddenly. Hatha Yoga commences with simple leg exercises, muscle stretching and the gradual and systematical practice of Asanas. Similarly, one must learn to master the breathing mechanism way in advance in order to consciously direct the Prana. That is why from the very beginning, Abdominal Breathing, Full Yogic Breath, Kapalabhati and Alternate Nostril Breathing should be performed.

6

IN ORDER TO PURIFY THE SUSHUMNA NADI, PRANAYAMA SHOULD BE PRACTICED DAILY WITH A SATTWIC STATE OF MIND.

The most important instruction concerning Pranayama is that it be done daily with a Sattwic state of mind. A focused mind is needed when doing breathing exercises. Whatever the state of mind, that is what will be magnified during Pranayama. When a person is in a positive state of mind, Pranayama will enhance that Sattwic state further. That peaceful state is reached when the mind is free from the lower nature of anger, lust, greed, hatred, jealousy, envy and fear. If on the other hand, a depressed or aggressive state persists, that degraded state is what will be magnified even more through Pranayama.

A Sattwic state of mind is obtained through positive thinking and observing Yamas and Niyamas. The practice of Asanas alone will not produce a Sattwic state of mind. A Sattwic mind cannot be induced instantly either. You cannot just turn on a switch of Sattwa. Instead, it has to be cultivated. Therefore, one can see the importance of observing the Yamas and Niyamas from the beginning of one's practice.

Many people have become experts in Yoga postures without having a Sattwic state of mind. They can still be hateful, greedy, envious and full of fear and egoism. A big time criminal could be a perfected Asana practitioner. Unless Yama and Niyama are observed and one lives, thinks and acts in a righteous manner, the mind will not become Sattwic.

That is why chanting the name of God and doing Japa are very helpful for restless people or for those who experience depression or anxiety. Chanting is very simple but ever so effective. Right association is of paramount importance. Regularity in practice is also critical. It is not sensible to practice Asana and Pranayama for a couple of hours on one day and then do nothing for the next few days because your body aches.

ANULOMA VILOMA
Alternate Nostril Breathing

7

SITTING IN PADMASANA, THE YOGI SHOULD INHALE THROUGH THE LEFT NOSTRIL AND HOLD THE BREATH TO HIS CAPACITY THEN EXHALE SLOWLY THROUGH THE RIGHT NOSTRIL.

8

THEN INHALING THROUGH THE RIGHT NOSTRIL AND HOLDING THE BREATH AS BEFORE, EXHALE SLOWLY AND COMPLETELY THROUGH THE LEFT NOSTRIL.

9

THUS BY INHALING THROUGH THE SAME NOSTRIL THAT THE BREATH WAS EXHALED, AND HOLDING THE BREATH TO CAPACITY, IT SHOULD BE EXHALED THROUGH THE OTHER NOSTRIL SLOWLY WITH CONTROL.

10
INHALE THROUGH THE LEFT NOSTRIL AND HOLDING THE BREATH TO CAPACITY, EXHALE THROUGH THE RIGHT. THEN INHALE THROUGH THE RIGHT AND RETAINING AS BEFORE, EXHALE THROUGH THE LEFT. BY PRACTICING IN THIS MANNER, THE YOGI GAINS PURITY OF THE NADIS WITHIN THREE MONTHS.

Anuloma Viloma or Alternate Nostril Breathing:

This is the Pranayama that further accelerates the purification of the Nadis, a process that began with observing Yama and Niyama, a moderate diet, the practice of Asanas and breathing exercises.

In the beginning, Alternate Nostril Breathing should be done at a very low ratio. The general rule is to respect a 1:4:2 ratio, the numbers referring to the counts of inhalation, retention and exhalation, respectively. If retaining the breath is too stressful in the beginning, one can start by alternately inhaling and exhaling through the separate nostrils as in Full Yogic Breathing but without holding the breath in between. Then continue as hereby instructed.

Technique: To prepare for the exercise, one sits in a comfortable position, with the back, neck and head in one vertical straight line. The right hand is held in Vishnu Mudra (index and middle fingers are bent) to close the right nostril with the thumb and the left with the ring finger. Begin the exercise with an exhalation. Close the right nostril with the thumb and start Anuloma Viloma by inhaling through the left nostril; hold the breath; exhale right; inhale right; hold the breath; exhale left. This completes one round. It is important that you do not count too fast and it is recommended that you tune into the heartbeat because this develops inner focus.

ANULOMA VILOMA

1
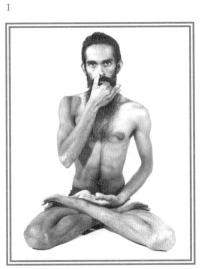

2
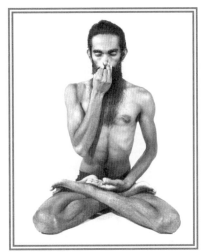

3
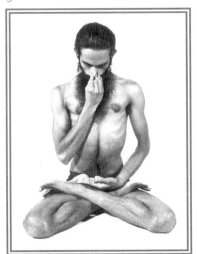

4
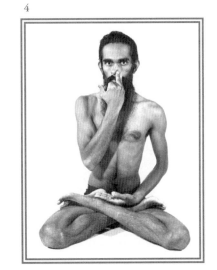

Retention with Bandhas

Practice for awhile with the count of 4:16:8 and do this for about 12 minutes at each sitting. Once this becomes comfortable, you can gradually increase the counts so long as you respect the ratio of 1:4:2. That is, inhale 5, retain 20, exhale 10. Then move on to inhale for 6, retain 24 and exhale 12. Inhale 7, retain 28 and exhale 14. Then inhale 8, retain 32 and exhale 16. Do not proceed to a higher count until the breathing becomes comfortable at each stage. Once you are able to practice according to the 8:32:16 count, there is no need to increase it any further. From then on, you just increase the number of rounds of Anuloma Viloma until you practice for a half an hour every sitting.

The practice of Alternate Nostril Breathing must be done systematically and without forcing. Different people have different capabilities. If you experience difficulty complying with the count, move back to a lower number until it becomes very comfortable. If you find yourself straining to hold the breath, you will not be able to have a controlled exhalation. That is why it is advisable to practice Pranayama according to the instructions of a Guru who can monitor your ability instead of blindly following the instructions in a book. Practicing without proper guidance can lead one to misinterpretation, cause unnecessary strain and discomfort, and deprive one of realizing the benefits of Pranayama altogether.

11
THIS PRACTICE SHOULD BE DONE FOUR TIMES DAILY: EARLY MORN-ING, MIDDAY, EVENING AND MIDNIGHT WITH THE RETENTION GRAD-UALLY INCREASED TO EIGHTY.

Instead of holding the breath up to 80 counts, I recommend that you retain up to 32 counts. The instruction to practice four times a day in order for purification to take place in three months is meant for the Yogi living in solitude. It is for the Sadhaka who is free from distractions, responsibilities and worries.

After having practiced Pranayama, wait half an hour before eating. Eat moderately and food that is easily digestible so that you can start your Pranayama again if you are practicing four times a day. This is the primary reason for observance of this special diet as prescribed in chapter 1.

> **12**
> **IN THE BEGINNING STAGE OF THE PRACTICE, THERE WILL BE PERSPIRATION. IN THE MIDDLE STAGE, THERE WILL BE TREMBLING AND IN THE FINAL STAGE, THERE WILL BE COMPLETE STILLNESS. THEREFORE, THE PRACTICE SHOULD CONTINUE UNTIL THIS FINAL STAGE IS REACHED.**

In the beginning of the purification process, one sweats when practicing Pranayama. People who take a Yoga class for the first time sweat profusely. Because of all the impurities, their sweat also reeks, depending on what they ate on that day and in prior years. In the middle stage, as you continue to progress, your body will tremble as a result of the purification process and the Prana attempting to move. In the final stage, when the body is completely purified, there is complete steadiness and stillness. That is when you experience the flow of Prana and peace.

These are the indications of the different stages of the Nadi purification. The sweating is the most obvious and prevalent in the beginning. Trembling is the intermediate stage. Some people revel in this stage mistaking the trembling as a sign of Kundalini awakening. That is far from the truth so do not get stuck in this delusion. Plod on with your practice until the final stage of stillness and bliss is experienced.

13

**THE PERSPIRATION THAT OCCURS THROUGH THE PRACTICE OF
PRANAYAMA SHOULD BE RUBBED BACK INTO THE BODY. THIS GIVES
FIRMNESS AND STEADINESS TO THE BODY.**

In the beginning, when the body is very toxic and the perspiration reeks, it is not
advisable to rub the sweat back in but to wipe it off instead. Once the body
becomes more purified and the sweat itself is pure, it is beneficial to rub it back
into the skin in order to recuperate the minerals and electrolytes that would otherwise be lost.

SUITABLE DIET FOR PRANAYAMA

14

**FOOD CONSISTING OF MILK AND GHEE IS RECOMMENDED IN THE
BEGINNING STAGE OF THE PRACTICE. WHEN ONE BECOMES ESTAB-
LISHED IN THE PRACTICE, SUCH RESTRICTIONS ARE NOT NECESSARY.**

The practice of Pranayama dries up the mucus in the body, which needs to be
replenished to avoid imbalance. When one experiences excessive heat while practicing Pranayama, it is useful to consume dairy products and observe a Yogic diet.

Some people recommend complete elimination of dairy products from one's diet
because they can provoke congestion. But this occurs in people who are not
involved in this kind of discipline. Dairy is not bad in itself. Its effect on people
depends on who uses it and for what purpose. Different people recommend different things. It all depends on your level of practice, your condition and your
constitution. To avoid confusion, listen to your Guru. Follow the advice of the
Scriptures written by Saints and Rishis who speak from experience.

15

JUST AS A LION, AN ELEPHANT OR A TIGER REQUIRES KNOWLEDGE, CARE AND PATIENCE TO TAME, SIMILARLY TO BRING THE PRANA UNDER CONTROL REQUIRES PROPER KNOWLEDGE, PATIENCE AND CARE OR ELSE THE PRACTITIONER IS DESTROYED.

It is very important to proceed with Pranayama in a careful, systematic and progressive way. Otherwise things might get out of hand. Problems might arise because the individual is not able to channel the energy. It could take years to restore the normal state. Taming a tiger presupposes the study of its character, habits, behavior and risk of aggression. If one approaches the animal unwittingly as if it were a sweet cat, one is surely in for a big surprise. Similarly, if one wants to control the Prana, its mechanisms must first be studied and the body and mind prepared. One must have proper knowledge and understanding and approach the practice with care and patience.

Some schools of Yoga cater to individuals who desire to skip the elementary stages and immediately dive into advanced techniques from the onset. There are some practices that introduce advanced breathing techniques like Bhastrika in the very beginning. This is dangerous for people who have an impure body and a disturbed state of mind.

16

ALL DISEASES CAN BE ERADICATED THROUGH THE PROPER PRACTICE OF PRANAYAMA WHILE IMPROPER PRACTICE CAN RESULT IN ALL SORTS OF PROBLEMS.

As discussed earlier, Prana nourishes the bodily systems and purifies the Nadis. It cleanses the lungs, heart and internal organs. Through a systematic practice of Pranayama, as outlined in the begining of this chapter, one can regain and maintain a vibrant state of health. This Sloka emphasizes the importance of right practice. A person of right discrimination seeks out a competent Guru for guidance so that he can practice with confidence.

17
HICCOUGH, ASTHMA, COUGH, PAIN IN THE HEAD, EAR AND EYES AND VARIOUS OTHER DISEASES ARE DUE TO VATA DISTURBANCE.

Ayurveda, the traditional Indian medicine and the Vedic science of healing, distinguishes three Doshas or constitutions, which operate at the level of body, mind and conciousness. The Doshas are known as Vata, Pitta and Kapha. The concept of the Tridosha in Ayurveda is unlike anything known in Western medicine. According to Ayurveda, the human body and the senses are manifestations of cosmic energy as the five elements: earth, water, fire, air and ether. Because these five elements exist in combinations in man, food and plants, the Rishis discovered that they could use food to regain and maintain balance and health. The combination of the five elements manifest in the body as the Tridoshas. Ayurveda strives to promote health through balancing the Tridoshas.

Vata governs all the body's biological movements, including breathing, blinking, nerve impulses and heart pulsation. Its elements are ether and air. Pitta governs the body's metabolism. Its elements are fire and water. People with a Pitta constitution generally have a good digestive fire. Kapha governs the bodily resistance, lubrication of the joints and the production of mucus. Its constituting elements are water and earth.

This Sloka lists various Vata disturbances. Because the elements of Vata are ether and air, which are related to the Vishuddi Chakra (throat Chakra) and the

Anahata Chakra (heart Chakra). Disturbances in the movement of Prana and Apana here can result in disease in the bronchial and vocal apparatus, lungs, alimentary canal, ears, nose, throat, heart, blood, vagus nerve and circulatory system. In addition, due to the air element, Vata's attributes are mobility, lightness, dryness and dispersion. Any of these qualities in excess will cause an imbalance of Vata while the opposite qualities will help to restore the balance. Moreover, since mobility, lightness and dryness predominate in the external environment during the fall season, Vata in the body will naturally be aggrevated during fall.

The science of Ayurveda can help you learn about your constitution, whether you are Vata, Pitta or Kapha. Then you will be able to know whether a certain Dosha is out of balance and modify your diet and lifestyle to help regain balance.

18
SUCCESS IN PRANAYAMA IS ATTAINED THROUGH SKILLFUL PRACTICE OF INHALATION, RETENTION AND EXHALATION.

The "skillful" practice of inhalation, retention and exhalation means a systematic approach, as described earlier. When you are able to perform Alternate Nostril Breathing according to the 8:32:16 count in a very comfortable way, you can start applying the Bandhas, which are Mula Bandha and Jalandhara Bandha during retention, and Uddiyana Bandha after exhalation. *(See Sloka 46 of this chapter for instructions on the Bandhas.)* In that case, you return to a basic count of 4:16:8 and apply the Bandhas because if you start the Bandhas at a count of 8:32:16, you will create undue stress in your system.

19

WHEN THE NADIS ARE PURIFIED, THE BODY BECOMES LEAN AND IT GLOWS. THESE ARE THE EXTERNAL SIGNS OF SUCCESS.

As the body purifies, external signs begin to show. The body of someone who practices Hatha Yoga will naturally normalize its weight. The face will appear younger and the body will glow with Prana and light of higher consciousness.

With Hatha Yoga, one really refines and purifies the body on a more subtle level. This is one of the main differences between Yoga, on the one hand, and weight lifting or fitness training, on the other hand, which do not refine the body.

Yoga restores balance in the body and induces all the systems to function more efficiently. It is also done for different purposes, mainly to raise consciousness, transform the personality and become more enlightened. This is simply not the goal in fitness training or weightlifting. A beautiful person with a well-shaped body can easily have a clouded consciousness and seem unanimated. In that case, his personality and face will still express base consciousness. On the other hand, a person who practices Yoga for liberation will not only have a beautiful physique, but his mind will also be at a higher level of consciousness, and therefore the entire body and face will reflect divinity. When the body and mind become purified, consciousness expresses in a pure state. Yoga works on the purification of the Nadis. But Nadis are not only physical channels. They also run through the energy, emotional and mental systems. As this purification takes place, it shows in one's face and personality.

20

WHEN THE NADIS ARE PURIFIED, THE BREATH IS RETAINED EASILY, THE DIGESTIVE POWER INCREASES, THE DIVINE SOUND IS AWAKENED AND ONE IS FREED FROM DISEASES.

These are more subtle signs of the purification of the Nadis. The more the Nadis become purified, the easier it becomes to retain the breath while performing Kumbhaka. In fact, one reaches a point where the breath is suspended. My Guru, Swami Nada Brahmananda suspended his breath for 37 minutes every morning, in the practice of Nada Kumbhaka. He was able to do this because his body was in a purified state, meaning the body was no longer purging so many toxins, thereby obviating the need for him to breathe in order to induce an exchange of toxins for pure air in the lungs. The Prana was also under control and the mind completely calm, resulting in less use of energy and the body's need for oxygen. On a lower level, one can experience how much easier it is to retain the breath in Pranayama when the mind is calm and peaceful. When there is agitation, retention becomes very strenuous.

People with a good digestive fire often make the mistake of thinking that they have to eat more to compensate. They mistakenly believe that they will lack nutrition. This is not true and certainly is not a reason to indulge in excessive food consumption. That would be an example of wrong discrimination. It would unnecessarily burden the body and deprive one of energy. With a moderate diet, the aspirant will benefit from swift digestion because he will be ready to continue his Sadhana shortly after eating a meal.

When the Nadis are purified and you sit quietly, you will experience the subtle vibrations of Prana, referred to as the Anahata Sound or the internal music. That will charm the mind to take you into a deeper state of awareness until that focus of mind eventually culminates in Samadhi. The Divine or Anahata sound does not have to be awakened. It is always there but can only be experienced when body and mind have been refined and purified.

SHATKRIYAS

21

**WHEN THERE IS EXCESS OF FAT AND MUCUS, THE SHATKRIYAS
SHOULD BE PRACTICED BEFORE PRANAYAMA. THOSE IN WHOM THE
DOSHAS ARE BALANCED, NEED NOT DO THEM.**

The Shatkriyas are cleansing techniques, sometimes referred to as the Shatkarmas.
There are six cleansing techniques in Hatha Yoga that are designed to help accelerate the cleansing process by removing the gross impurities. This cleansing takes place
on different levels, including the physical, emotional, mental and intellectual.

When we become involved in Hatha Yoga, we become more aware of our body
and begin to understand the enormous amount of impurities that we somehow
managed to accumulate over many years. Usually, people are totally ignorant of
this fact, and therefore impurities continue to amass until the person reaches a cri-
sis situation. That is when he will visit a doctor, get a prescription and take medicine, which in turn will only mask the symptoms.

The Shatkriyas are the main facilitator for healing. Usually when people feel their
body stagnating, they immediately think of which medicine to take, which only
creates more congestion. Whereas, Hatha Yoga and natural healing concentrate
on eliminating toxins, freeing the body of congestion and stimulating the natural functioning of the body through exercise, proper diet, Pranayama, positive
thinking, etc.

In Yogic practices, you become more aware of your body and begin to understand that
the process of refinement helps you to develop increased awareness of the Self. This
self-awareness naturally starts with the body since that is what you can relate to more
easily. Next, you become aware of your emotions, your energy system, your mind, etc.

This self-awareness alerts you to the malfunctions in the body's systems so that they can be corrected with Asanas, Pranayama and proper diet before they develop into more health problems.

In Hatha Yoga, you learn about the importance of positive thinking along with the practice of Asanas and breathing exercises, which deepens your connection to your body. You will begin to experience limitations in the body, including flexibilty, strength, stamina and blockages in the flow of energy. When you start doing breathing exercises, you may at first experience a great deal of mucus and congestion, which hampers proper breathing. You may also find that while doing Yoga, you experience some discomfort in your stomach or intestines and realize that you have been constipated for a long time.

People experience ill health, obesity, congestion, light headedness and other conditions because the Doshas are not in balance. When there is imbalance in the body, whether it be Vata, Pitta or Kapha, the body will constantly struggle to regain balance. When there is balance, the body does not have to struggle, thereby freeing the mind to contemplate and experience the higher reality. The Shatkarmas are very effective in helping to bring about balance in the Doshas. They will free one from mucus and obesity by regulating and increasing the efficient functioning of the bodily systems such as the digestive, respiratory, circulatory, endocrine, nervous and elimination systems.

The Shatkriyas are done when the body shows an excess in the Tridoshas. It is not necessary to wait until Asana practice has been perfected before applying the Shatkriyas but there must be a certain bodily awareness. After having reached a certain level in the practice of Asanas and breathing exercises, the body may struggle to breathe or show congestion. That is when the practice of the Kriyas can be started. An enema is particularly recommended while fasting so that the released toxins can be purged faster and the purification process can be enhanced.

When the Doshas are balanced and you have reached a certain level of purity and awareness, the Shatkriyas will no longer be necessary. By then, one will be living a disciplined life and observing a moderate diet so that the body does not accumulate waste anymore. However, you can still do them once in a while for maintenance purposes.

22
THE SHATKRIYAS OR SIX CLEANSING EXERCISES ARE DHAUTI, BHASTI, NETI, NAULI, KAPALABHATI AND TRATAKA.

Yogis have prescribed six cleansing techniques that accelerate cleansing on the gross level. Vamana Dhauti is the cleansing of the stomach. Bhasti is the cleansing of the colon. Neti cleanses the nostrils and sinuses. Nauli is a manipulation of the abdominal muscles. It tones up the colon and abdominal viscera and removes sluggishness of the stomach, intestines and liver. The strengthening of the abdominal muscles assists in proper breathing. At a more subtle level, Nauli helps to sublimate the sexual energy, transforming it into mental energy. Kapalabhati is the cleansing of the lungs. It also strengthens the diaphragm and removes spasms in the bronchial tubes. Trataka is the cleansing of the eyes and nervous system. The techniques for each are described in subsequent Slokas.

23
THE YOGI DERIVES WONDERFUL BENEFITS FROM THESE SHATKRIYAS
AND THEY SHOULD ONLY BE GIVEN TO THOSE WHO ARE READY.

It is important to be secretive about your practice of the Shatkriyas because people who are just spectators may express disgust. They will shy away from you
because they are not mentally or emotionally ready. You also need to learn how to
do them properly from a Guru. People who do not have the necessary faith in
their Guru will not understand or learn the correct methods. If they see you doing
the Shatkriyas, such as swallowing a cloth or pushing a string through your nose
and pulling it out again from your mouth, they most likely would think that you
are crazy. You would become a side show, something that they would go to see in
a circus.

Some people get carried away by the practice and perform the Kriyas to demonstrate their own prowess. For example, a televison program showed a man doing
Neti with a small snake. He would guide the snake through his nose and direct it
through his mouth. When he was asked how long it took to accomplish that, he
answered 15 years.

Foolish practices like this give people the wrong idea of the purpose of Yoga. Some
Yogis are admired simply because they have mastered the Kriyas. When people
tout themselves as masters of such practices, it is most likely serving their own
egos, demonstrating pride and thereby straying from the real spirit of Yoga.
Everything must be practiced for a higher purpose.

D H A U T I

24

ONE SHOULD SWALLOW SLOWLY A WET PIECE OF CLOTH FOUR FINGERS IN WIDTH AND FIFTEEN CUBITS IN LENGTH AND TAKE IT OUT SLOWLY AS INSTRUCTED BY THE GURU. THIS IS KNOWN AS DHAUTI.

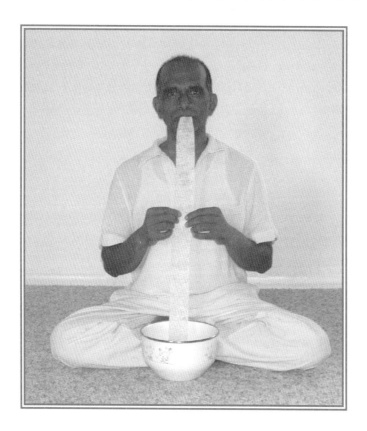

Dhauti is the cleansing of the stomach. There are two ways to do Dhauti: with cloth or water. If you opt for the cloth method, use sterile gauze about 4 fingers wide and place it in a bowl of lukewarm water. Do not fold the cloth. Keep a glass of lukewarm water handy so that you can take sips of water when necessary. Sit in a squatting position. To be able to swallow a long piece of cloth, you must alternately chew, swallow and drink some water. Eventually the throat will relax so that you can keep swallowing until you have nearly eaten the whole cloth. Make sure you keep a piece in your hand so that you will be able to gently take it back out. Resist the urge to vomit. Do not pull the cloth out suddenly or the epiglottis will contract because the peristaltic action there is not accustomed to something coming up. The first time I practiced Dhauti in this way, the cloth got stuck, which was a difficult situation to say the least. I had to consciously relax or I would have damaged my throat. Therefore, do not tense up when you do this cleansing exercise. Stay relaxed. You should also do this under the direction of a Guru so that you learn to do it properly.

The other way to perform Dhauti is to drink 4 to 8 glasses of saline water until your stomach is completely filled. The mixture is two teaspoons of salt to a quart of lukewarm water. Every time you gulp down a glass, you either do Nauli or jump up and down. You can also perform Uddhiyana Bandha. When you feel the stomach is full, put your index and middle fingers to the back of the throat and induce the gagging effect to vomit the water. Do not stop once you have started the vomiting or else you will have to reinstate it again and again. Continue until it feels as if your stomach is coming out.

To prepare for Dhauti, you could practice the vomiting action every morning by massaging your throat with the middle and index fingers until you get accustomed to gagging. It actually massages and strengthens the stomach. If you do that for a week or two before you perform Dhauti, you will become accustomed to that effect.

25

THERE IS NO DOUBT THAT BY PRACTICING DHAUTI, COUGH, ASTHMA, DISEASE OF THE SPLEEN, LEPROSY AND TWENTY KINDS OF DISEASES CAUSED BY EXCESS KAPHA ARE CURED.

Kapha governs the bodily resistance, lubrication of the joints and production of mucus. The seat of Kapha is in the chest. An imbalance in this Dosha may manifest as obesity, bronchitis or edema, for example. Dhauti is such a powerful cleansing technique that it can eradicate common illnesses resulting from infectious bacteria that cause coughing, asthma, and serious diseases such as leprosy.

Dhauti cleanses the entire digestive and respiratory tracts, purges mucus, old excess bile and toxins and restores the chemical composition of the body to its natural balanced state. It also eliminates infectious bacteria from the mouth, nose, eyes, ears, throat, stomach, intestines and anus. It reduces excess fat and alleviates chronic flatulence, constipation, poor digestion and loss of appetite. Dhauti can cure abdominal ailments and fever but it is important not to practice Dhauti while you are running a fever or if you have an acute infection. Once you regain your health, the practice of Dhauti can help to prevent the recurrence of that same illness.

B H A S T I

26

SQUATTING NAVEL DEEP IN CLEAN WATER, INSERT A TUBE INTO THE ANUS AND THROUGH CONTRACTION, PULL THE WATER UP INTO THE COLON. THIS WASHING IS CALLED BHASTI.

Bhasti is the cleansing of the colon. This Sloka instructs how to do Bhasti according to the traditional method, which would create many problems today because there are no clean rivers any more. You would be insane to squat in a polluted river. Instead, you could sit in a tub of water. Back then, one used to take a piece of hollow bamboo about 4 inches in length, lubricate it and insert it into the anus. Then one would practice Uddiyana Bandha and Nauli to create a vacuum in the intestines, thus drawing water into the colon. Once the water had been drawn in, the tube would be removed. Then one would repeat Nauli and expel the water. The action of releasing out and drawing in water was repeated until the whole colon was cleansed.

Today, it is sufficient to take an enema. Most people either have never heard about an enema or cringe at the thought of using it. Why would someone think it is disgusting to wash their colon? It is simply a case of wrong conditioning. When we get up in the morning or when we finish eating a meal, we brush our teeth without even thinking about it. We just do it. This is normal, acceptable behavior because when it is not done, the mouth emits a foul odor. Yet most people find washing the rest of the alimentary canal disgusting. The digestive tract consists of the mouth, pharynx, esophagus, stomach, intestines, colon and anus. The entire structure of the digestive tract needs to be cleansed from time to time. If one neglects parts of it, ultimately, one may develop cancer of the colon or other diseases.

It is important to note that the alimentary canal is a muscular tube that runs through the body. That is why it needs to be kept clean. This is the part of the digestive system where food is processed. The nutrients are then absorbed into the bloodstream. Everything else, which is the waste, passes through and is eliminated.

The large intestine does not secrete any digestive juices. The body simply reabsorbs water from the intestinal contents and eliminates the solid waste through the anal canal. If proper elimination does not occur, toxins and waste products continue to accumulate for years in the large intestine, which becomes a breeding ground for disease and all kinds of health problems. Therefore, it is important to make sure that your alimentary canal is clean and working properly. This includes the colon.

27
THROUGH THE PRACTICE OF BHASTI, ENLARGEMENT OF THE GLANDS AND SPLEEN AND DISEASES ARISING FROM EXCESS OF VATA, PITTA AND KAPHA ARE ELIMINATED.

28
BHASTI INCREASES THE APPETITE, BALANCES THE DOSHAS, PURIFIES THE DHATUS, SENSES AND MIND AND MAKES THE BODY GLOW.

Many problems are created because of congestion in the intestines. When autopsies are performed, in some cases, they find up to twenty pounds of feces still in the body. This means that it has been accumulating and caking there for years, preventing proper absorption of nutrients. This also results in inflammation of the intestines. It is a process analogous to the calcification and occlusion of water pipes. You can see now why cleansing of the colon is so important.

Through the practice of Bhasti, your appetite will increase, and because everything will be flowing and functioning properly, the body will glow.

Due to interaction with the external environment and to cultural and social conditioning, imbalance occurs in the harmonious functioning of the Doshas. This, in turn, affects the Dhatus, the seven vital tissues of the body, and the Srotas (Nadis), the subtle channels through which the energy flows, thereby creating Ama, the waste accumulated through poor digestion and absorption. This, in turn, may result in disease. Bhasti purifes the Dhatus and balances the Doshas, the senses and the mind.

Health does not only relate to the physical body. What happens at the physical level is most often the reflection of what happens at a subtle level, and vice-versa. Hatha Yoga teaches that we have three bodies and five sheaths. The physical body is the Annamaya Kosha or the food sheath. So when people say, "You are what you eat," that is really true. The Astral body consists of the Pranamaya Kosha or the energy sheath, the Manomaya Kosha or the mental sheath, and the Vijnanamaya Kosha or the intellect sheath. Finally, you have the causal body, which is the Anandamaya Kosha or the blissful sheath. The three bodies and the five sheaths are the instruments through which the soul experiences the world. Therefore, whatever happens on one sheath affects the other sheaths. When one practices the Shatkriyas, one establishes integration on all levels of one's being, including the physical, emotional, mental, psychic and cosmic.

The practice of Bhasti cleanses the physical body and therefore affects the more subtle layers. Physical tensions reflect mental tensions. When people are constipated, their mind is also constipated. They suffer from sluggishness, laziness, Tamas and headaches. The moment that person goes to the bathroom, he will be so relieved that he will be smiling at everything. It is very painful to do Asanas and Pranayama properly when you are constipated. Freedom in the limbs, high energy and harmony in the body naturally develop a feeling of joy and happiness. Therefore, as soon as constipation is relieved, the mind will be clear and that person will really enjoy Asana. It is a very practical way of purification. When the body is purified, the mind will stabilize and responses to situations that normally induce exaggerated emotional reactions will subside. One will respond in a more relaxed and deliberate way because everything is in balance.

It is important to note that if you do not have constipation, it is sufficient to take an enema only once in awhile, maybe every few months.

N E T I

29

INSERT A CHORD MADE OF THREAD ABOUT NINE INCHES LONG THROUGH THE NOSE AND PULL IT OUT THROUGH THE MOUTH. THIS IS NETI.

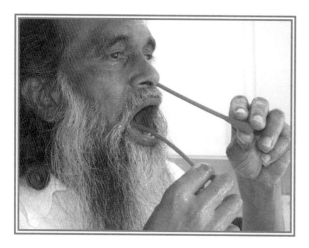

Sutra Neti

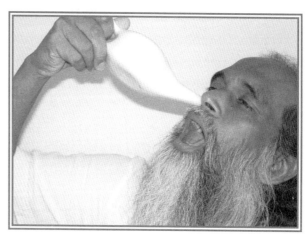

Jala Neti

Neti is the cleansing of the nostrils and sinuses either with a string or catheter, which is known as Sutra Neti, or with lukewarm water, which is known as Jala Neti. Neti stimulates the circulation, drains mucus and creates a healthy nasal area and sinuses. This is important because there are receptors of Prana in the nostrils.

According to the traditional methods of practicing Sutra Neti, Yogis used to take a thread, fold it many times and put wax on the end in order to make a stiff tip so that it would be possible to insert it in the nose. Today, a catheter is used instead. As you insert the catheter, you will find a passage up the nose where the catheter goes through and then down into the throat. It is important to stay relaxed while doing this. Do not push the catheter through with force. Instead, gently push it as it drops down into the throat area. Grab it there with two fingers, pull it out a bit and floss the nose. Repeat the process in the other nostril.

You can also practice Jala Neti using water. It is a very simple process. You take some water in your hand and pour it down both nostrils. The water should come out the mouth when you do this. This is especially helpful when you are traveling and feel tired. Go to the rest stop, wash your face, take some water in your hand and pour it down both nostrils. This will wake you up again. Some people use a special Neti Lota or Neti Pot that is designed to fit into the nostril. The truth is that you will get the same effect if you just use your hands to pour water down the nostrils. Then you will not need any special equipment. Jala Neti can be done every time you brush your teeth or wash your face.

Whatever means you use, after you have finished Neti, you will feel very clean, invigorated and clear. You will also be able to do Pranayama very nicely.

30

NETI CLEANSES THE BRAIN AND BESTOWS CLAIRVOYANCE. IT ALSO DESTROYS ALL DISEASES ABOVE THE SHOULDERS.

Neti alleviates sinus congestion, dryness in the nose, a hoarse throat, tonsillitis, migraine headaches, certain eye and ear infections, colds, allergies and even convulsions. The nasal cavity filters bacteria and dust, and the blood from the capillaries warms and moistens the air on its way to the lungs. The absence of moisture can destroy the cilia, which are the little hairs in the lining of the respiratory tract that assist in filtering dust particles. By stimulating and washing out the nasal area with water through the practice of Neti, eliminates accumulated bacteria and mucus in the nostrils. Jala Neti also helps to moisten a dry nose. All of this, in turn, allows the air to flow unobstructed.

The olfactory nerve in the nasal cavity functions as the sense of smell. The bulb of the nerve goes right into the brain so that you can sense poisons before they are inhaled. There are tiny paired cavities (spaces) in the bony structure of the skull called the sinuses, which are also lined with mucous membranes for cleansing of inspired air. These sinuses also serve as sound chambers giving us resonance. Neti promotes the drainage of these sinuses and alleviates accumulated mucus, which naturally has a positive effect on the ears, eyes, nose and throat.

Since receptors of Prana are also in the nose, Neti will also help to alleviate disorders of Prana that affect the higher cerebral, sensory and motor functions, which include, among other things, speech, language, abstract reasoning, hearing, emotions, memory and vision. When Prana is flowing evenly through both nostrils, the left and right hemispheres of the brain will be balanced, the bodily systems will be harmonized and one will experience peace and tranquility. The practice of Neti also stimulates the Ajna Chakra, the third eye, the seat of consciousness, because it removes blockages and allows for the free flow of Prana. This is why it is said that Neti bestows clairvoyance.

TRATAKA

31
GAZE AT A POINT WITHOUT BLINKING, WITH THE EYES RELAXED, UNTIL TEARS FLOW. THIS IS TRATAKA.

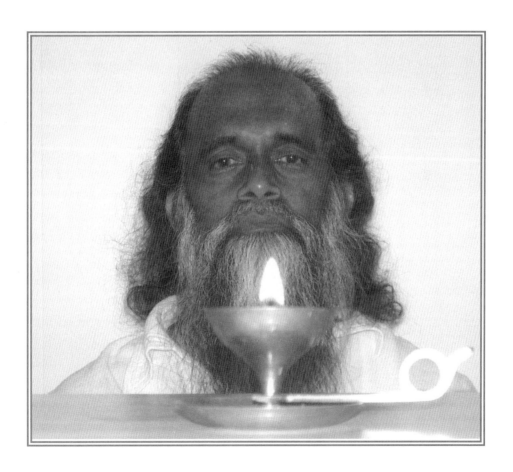

Trataka cleans and strengthens the eyes and nervous system. It also greatly develops concentration. Trataka on the flame of a candle has to be done in a windless place about 7 to 10 feet away from the candle. The flame has to be steady and level with your eyes. Sit up straight, keep the eyes, body and mind relaxed. Gaze at the flame without straining the eyes or blinking. You can do this for about five minutes. Then close your eyes and visualize the flame at the point between your eyebrows. You can mentally repeat your Mantra, and if you do not have a Mantra, then you can repeat "Om." This will bring your mind to a state of peace.

The flame is a powerful symbol of the inner light but Trataka is done only for concentration purposes. Instead of a flame, you can use a simple dot as the point of concentration.

32
TRATAKA REMOVES FATIGUE, SLOTH AND EYE DISEASES. IT SHOULD BE VALUED JUST AS ONE WOULD VALUE A CASKET OF GOLD.

Trataka also bestows clairvoyance and the ability to read auras. If you stare at a candle flame without blinking, you will begin to notice the subtle aura around the flame. Trataka is performed with relaxed eyes. When you use a soft gaze, you are using the rods rather than the cones in your eyes, which enables you to see auras.

Since the mind is usually scattered, it pulls you in many different directions, thereby depleting your energy. By focusing attention on one object, the vacillating nature of the mind eventually ceases and the power of the mind increases. Thus, Trataka helps to eliminate fatigue normally produced by the wandering mind. The practice of Trataka also improves eyesight and stimulates the brain through the optic nerve.

N A U L I

33

LEAN FORWARD AND PLACE THE HANDS ON THE KNEES. PROTRUDE THE ABDOMEN AND ROTATE THE MUSCLES FROM RIGHT TO LEFT WITH SPEED LIKE A STRONG WHIRLPOOL. THIS IS NAULI.

Nauli is a manipulation of the abdominal muscles. It tones up the colon and abdominal viscera, removes sluggishness of the stomach, intestines and liver. The strengthening of the abdominal muscles assists in proper breathing. At a more subtle level, Nauli helps to sublimate the sexual energy, transforming it into mental energy. The spiritual path requires a lot of energy and mental power and Nauli enhances this process.

Nauli starts from Uddiyana Bandha. Before you can perform Nauli, you must practice Uddiyana Bandha regularly for a few weeks. Perform Uddiyana Bandha before you begin your daily Asana practice. This enables you to gain a certain degree of control over the abdominal muscles, tones and strengthens the reproductive organs and helps to force Prana up the Sushumna Nadi.

Technique for Uddiyana Bandha:

In a standing position bend forward and place the hands firmly on the knees with the legs apart about two feet. Forcibly exhale the breath completely. At the end of the exhalation, pull the abdomen in and up towards the spine. Hold it for awhile and keep that position as long as the breath is held out. Then release the abdomen and inhale slowly with control. Then exhale completely and repeat the action. After a few weeks, the muscles will become nicely toned and strengthened.

NAULI

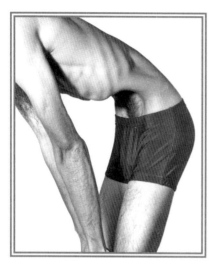

Uddiyana Bandha

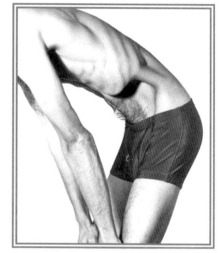

Nauli

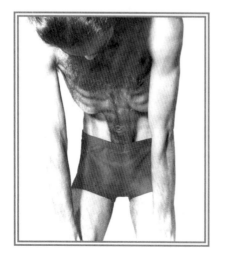

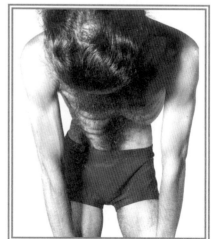

Technique for Nauli

At that stage, you protrude the muscles through concentration. It will happen naturally. Take the muscles to one side and then to the other side. Keep moving them from side to side in a churning motion. Rotate in a clockwise direction and then in the opposite direction.

> **34**
> **NAULI IS HELD IN HIGH ESTEEM IN HATHA YOGA PRACTICE. IT INCREASES THE DIGESTIVE FIRE, REMOVES DISORDERS OF THE DOSHAS AND BRINGS ABOUT HAPPINESS.**

The body has an innate intelligence. But if you do not listen to the body, its natural rhythm and harmony will deteriorate. If there is balance in the Doshas, you will experience health. On the other hand, when there is an imbalance in the Doshas, you will become sick. You will recall that the Doshas are Vata, Pitta and Kapha, which relate to different constitutions. The seat of Vata is the colon; the seat of Pitta is the stomach and small intestine; and the seat of Kapha is the chest. If there is derangement and imbalance in the Doshas, you must take certain precautions and implement certain practices to restore the balance.

The science of Hatha Yoga, when properly practiced, is a divine gift that restores balance and harmony to the three bodies and five sheaths. Nauli is very effective in removing disorders of the Doshas because as you manipulate the abdominal muscles, you are actually massaging the internal organs of the digestive tract and the reproductive system. Nauli helps the alimentary canal function properly. Therefore, it helps to reinstate the body's innate intelligence. And as discussed earlier, when your gastro intestinal tract is functioning properly, you feel healthy and happy.

KAPALABHATI

35

PERFORM EXHALATION FORCEFULLY AND WHEN RELEASED INHALATION TAKES PLACE NATURALLY. DOING THIS IN QUICK SUCCESSION LIKE THE BELLOWS OF A BLACKSMITH IS CALLED KAPALABHATI AND IT DESTROYS ALL MUCUS DISORDERS.

Kapalabhati is the cleansing of the lungs. It strengthens the diaphragm and removes spasm in the bronchial tubes.

Technique for Kapalabhati

To do Kapalabhati properly, sit up straight and keep your chest and shoulders relaxed. Only the diaphragm and abdominal muscles will be contracted as you forcefully exhale. Then let go and let the air rush in again. When you finish a round of expulsions, take a deep breath and at the same time, energize the body by stretching the arms out to the sides at shoulder level, making movements with the hands to release tensions. Exhale completely while bringing the arms down. Then inhale and retain the breath. Start with three rounds: the first round comprising twenty expulsions; the second, thirty expulsions; and the third, forty expulsions. Retain the breath for thirty seconds in the first round, forty-five seconds in the second round, and finish with one minute in the third round. The number of expulsions and length of breath retentions can be gradually increased to whatever count you want.

Anybody can do Kapalabhati. The forced exhalation is comparable to blowing your nose.

Contrary to Bhastrika where you inhale and exhale forcefully, in Kapalabhati, the emphasis is on the exhalation only, and the inhalation happens naturally as a result of the vacuum that has been created in the lungs.

Health invariably leads to happiness. But to experience this, the body must be cleansed of toxins, the mind must be steady and peaceful, the emotions must be calm and joyful, the body's wastes must be properly eliminated and the organs must be functioning properly and efficiently. The Kriyas are preventative activities that will help you attain this state. Most people would not understand these practices unless they have a Guru to teach them.

36
BY THE PRACTICE OF THE SHATKRIYAS, THE GROSS IMPURITIES ARE REMOVED AND THE DOSHAS ARE BALANCED. THEN THE PRACTICE OF PRANAYAMA BECOMES SUCCESSFUL WITHOUT STRAIN.

If the body is clogged with gross impurities and congested with excess mucus, you will be uncomfortable and straining to do breathing exercises. But once you practice the Shatkriyas and the gross impurities are removed, you will find the practice of Pranayama much easier and enjoyable. When you start to do Pranayama at this point, you will experience its cleansing effect and notice how still the mind becomes when you are finished.

Before starting Pranayama, you should have already included breathing exercises in your Asana practice. These include deep Abdominal Breathing, Full Yogic Breath, Kapalabhati and Alternate Nostril Breathing, performed as instructed at the beginning of this chapter.

37

**SOME ACHARIAS ADVOCATE THAT SINCE PRANAYAMA ALONE CAN
REMOVE THE IMPURITIES, THERE IS NO NEED FOR OTHER PRACTICES.**

Some teachers discourage people from practicing these cleansing techniques, advising students to simply perform Pranayama since that alone purifies the Nadis. The underlying reason for this is that many people become involved in practices without really knowing what they are doing. For them, it is often just a short lived fad for them to try. Without proper guidance and proper understanding, they can create a lot of problems for themselves. Doing something just for the sake of it in this case is not wise. It has to be done with a purpose. If you do not suffer from an excess of mucus, why would you want to do the Kriyas? Pranayama will be possible in that case because there is no blockage and therefore no need for Kriyas. Other people can only breathe through their mouth not through their nose. In fact, most people breathe through only one nostril. Normally, every few hours the other nostril takes over breathing. This is actually an indication that the Nadis are not purified. In the extreme case, people who use their nose to snort cocaine burn up all the mucous membranes in the process. They are destroying the innate intelligence of their body and creating all sorts of havoc.

GAJA KARANI

38

THE HATHA YOGI WITH KNOWLEDGE AND CONTROL CAN MOVE THE APANA VAYU TO THE THROAT AND VOMIT THE CONTENTS OF THE STOMACH. THIS IS GAJA KARANI.

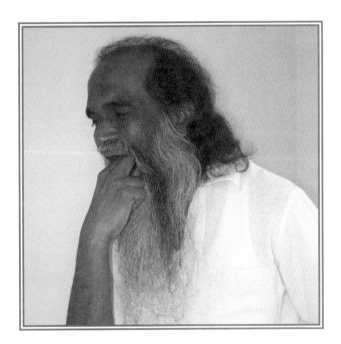

This practice is practical for the Yogi who is involved in this intense Sadhana doing Pranayama four times a day. You have to be very careful with this technique or it will lead to bulemia. Gaja Karani should not be practiced at any random time and certainly not after every meal. It should only be done according to the instructions of a Guru. After allowing a couple of hours for the food to digest, the remains in the stomach can be vomited back out. This way the body does not have to spend too much energy on processing the food. Only the essence of it is absorbed and the rest is discarded.

People who are not involved in this intense Sadhana can practice Gaja Karani only once in awhile, especially if you eat very heavy foods. When you ingest disagreeable food and your stomach becomes upset, it is very beneficial to regurgitate it, otherwise you will be suffering all night.

People often say "I have a bad stomach." But the truth is that your stomach is not bad, rather it is what you put into it. Since your body has an innate intelligence, it will inform you when you eat something bad. In this case, it is the stomach that is upset with you. However, most times we suppress that intelligence. We take medicines to mask that feeling, so that after awhile, our bodies no longer inform us. The disagreeable food will just pass through and create all sorts of problems in the body.

When you reach a certain level of purification, you become acutely aware of foods that are disagreeable. Once you reinstate that natural intelligence, your body will tell you.

It is similar to smoking for the first time and coughing. When you drink liquor for the first time, it burns as if it were firewater running down your throat. But if you continue smoking and drinking, that intelligence and sensibility is suppressed, and the body will cease alerting you. It becomes confused. So listen to the body when it talks to you.

39

EVEN BRAHMA AND THE OTHER GODS IN HEAVEN ARE DEVOTED TO THE PRACTICE OF PRANAYAMA BECAUSE IT ENDS THE FEAR OF DEATH. THEREFORE ONE SHOULD PRACTICE PRANAYAMA.

By indicating that even Brahma and the gods in heaven practice Pranayama, this Sloka tries to encourage you to do the same. Fear of death is one of the biggest fears people have. As a result, they resort to doing all kinds of nonsensical things, such as obsessively trying to preserve their bodies. Fear of death is one of the Kleshas, which are obstacles to enlightenment.

Pranayama will destroy the fear of death. Through this practice, the mind becomes steady and you experience more peace. As a result, you move away from body-consciousness to identify with the Higher Self more and more. This in turn, alleviates and ultimately dispels the fear of death. While you remain attached to the body and identify with it, you will always experience that trauma.

40

AS LONG AS THE BREATH IS RETAINED, THE MIND IS CALM AND THE GAZE IS CENTERED ON AJNA CHAKRA, WHY SHOULD THERE BE FEAR OF DEATH?

Fear of death vanishes once you have been able to experience your Higher Self. Once you really know that you are the Atman, the soul, you will not identify with this perishable body anymore and death will become irrelevant. Especially when the body becomes decrepit and you are suffering discomfort, you will gladly want to discard it.

41

WHEN THE NADIS AND CHAKRAS ARE PURIFIED THROUGH THE SYSTEMATIC PRACTICE OF PRANAYAMA, THE PRANA BURSTS OPEN THE DOORWAY TO SUSHUMNA AND EASILY ENTERS IT.

Sushumna is the most important Nadi to be purified. Through the systematic practice of Pranayama, the Nadis become purified and the Prana starts to flow through Sushumna, which will lead you to experience the unitive state and peace.

It is important to practice Pranayama correctly because it can create an imbalance in the body and mind if done incorrectly. As discussed earlier, whatever your state of mind is at the time, the practice of Pranayama will magnify it. So if you are in a depressed state, Pranayama could exacerbate that state. Therefore, you should only practice according to the instructions of a competent and knowlegable Guru.

MANONMANI

42

WHEN THE PRANA FLOWS THROUGH SUSHUMNA, THE MIND BECOMES STEADY. THIS STEADINESS OF MIND IS CALLED MANONMANI OR NO MIND.

Through the systematic practice of Asana and Pranayama, along with observing a Sattwic diet and living a simple secluded life without any distraction, the mind becomes steady. That is a result of the Nadis being purified and the Prana flowing through Sushumna.

The Ida and Pingala Nadis are a pair of opposites, positive and negative poles that induce fluctuations in energy. So long as the Prana is moving through either the Ida or Pingala Nadis, as they do in most people, one will be subject to experiencing duality, opposite polarities such as pain and joy, good and bad, etc. But when the Sushumna becomes purified and Prana flows through this middle passage, the mind becomes steady. That steadiness of mind is referred to as Manonmani, a mind devoid of thought.

43
TO ACHIEVE THIS, VARIOUS KUMBHAKAS ARE PERFORMED. THIS RESULTS IN VARIOUS SIDDHIS.

Kumbhakas are various breathing techniques to restrain and hold the breath. They help to accelerate the awakening of Kundalini Shakti and dormant parts of the brain. Through these practices, Siddhis or extraordinary powers are obtained.

KUMBHAKAS

44
THERE ARE EIGHT KUMBHAKAS. THESE ARE SURYABHEDA, UJJAYI, SITKARI, SITALI, BHASTRIKA, BHRAMARI, MURCHHA AND PLAVINI.

The methods and techniques of performing these eight specific Kumbhakas are described hereafter.

45
JALANDHARA BANDHA AND MULA BANDHA ARE DONE AT THE END OF INHALATION AND UDDIYANA BANDHA IS DONE AFTER EXHALATION.

46
THE PRANA WILL FLOW THROUGH THE BRAHMA NADI WHEN MULA BANDHA, JALANDHARA BANDHA AND UDDIYANA BANDHA ARE APPLIED.

Through these practices, eventually the Prana will flow through the Brahma Nadi, which is the Sushumna.

MULA BANDHA

To perform Mula Bandha, contract the perenium muscles. These are located in the area between the anus and the genetals. It is not to be confused with contraction of the anus, for this is another Mudra called Aswini Mudra. Mula Bandha takes dedicated practice to master but it bestows many benefits. It makes direct contact with Muladhara Chakra. When it is applied with Kumbhaka, it prevents Apana from escaping from the lower body. Instead, it draws the Apana upward to unite with Prana. This Mudra can also be applied in Asana practice, especially the standing postures, to give stability and improve concentration.

JALANDHARA BANDHA

To perform Jalandhara Bandha, while retaining the breath after inhalation, seal the tongue on the roof of the palate and press your chin firmly toward the chest and with the eyes closed, gaze at the point between the eyebrows. This prevents the Prana from escaping from the upper body.

UDDIYANA BANDHA

To perform Uddiyana Bandha, after exhaling, pull the abdomen up and toward the spine. This forces Prana up the Sushumna Nadi. *For more on these Bandhas, see chapter 3, Verses 55 to 78.*

47

BY RAISING THE APANA UP AND FORCING THE PRANA DOWN FROM THE THROAT, THE YOGI BECOMES FREE OF OLD AGE AND APPEARS LIKE A YOUTH OF SIXTEEN.

This is a very mystical teaching. When you gain a certain degree of awareness and control over the Prana, you can store it, redirect it and use it where and when it is needed, which results in a revitalization of the body and a general appearance of youthfulness.

Within the individual, the lifeforce or Prana is divided into 5 categories according to its function. These are referred to as the Pancha Prana. They are Prana, Apana, Samana, Vyana and Udana.

Prana functions in the system of perception. The individual is nourished not only by physical food and liquid taken in through the mouth, but also by everything taken in through the senses. Therefore, in conjunction with observing proper diet, you have to be discriminative as to what enters through the senses. You can be enriched or polluted by the things you hear. If you listen to Divine music or discourses from the Scriptures about God from your Guru or Saints, your mind and body will be nourished and purified. Whereas, if you listen to gossip and degrading music, your consciousness will be degraded. It is the same with all the other senses. Life can be made joyful, happy and youthful if you are aware and exercise right discrimination and dispassion as to what enters the system.

Forcing Prana down means to exercise control of the inward flow of energy. Do not take in everything without right discrimination. Exercise discipline of the senses and avoid overindulgence.

Raising Apana up is to be aware of what is thrown out and when. Apana functions in the organs of elimination, causing things to be thrown out of the system. This includes spit, stool, urine, perspiration, exhalation, the reproductive seed, etc. However you do not want to "throw out the baby with the bath water." For example, you do not want to bleed when there is no wound, as in hemmoroids. You do not want the sexual energy flowing out indiscriminately. And you do not want to suffer from diarrhea. This could also include excessive talking.

So to raise Apana up is to sublimate the sexual energy so that Ojas, Tejas and Prana is increased. This is a sure way to be free from old age and to maintain youthfulness.

SURYABHEDA

48

SIT IN A COMFORTABLE POSTURE, INHALE THROUGH THE RIGHT NOSTRIL.

49

RETAIN THE BREATH UNTIL IT FEELS LIKE IT IS DIFFUSING TO THE ROOT OF THE HAIR AND THE TIPS OF THE NAILS. THEN EXHALE SLOWLY THROUGH THE LEFT NOSTRIL.

50

SURYABHEDA IS EXCELLENT FOR PURIFYING THE CRANIUM, CORRECTING VATA IMBALANCE AND ELIMINATING WORMS. IT SHOULD BE PRACTICED AGAIN AND AGAIN.

"Surya" means "sun" and refers to the Pingala Nadi, which is governed by the right nostril. "Bheda" means "to pierce." The practice of Suryabheda pierces the Pingala Nadi, thereby activating Prana Shakti and generating heat in the body.

In Suryabheda, always inhale slowly through the right nostril, closing the left nostril with the ring finger of your right hand, which is held in Vishnu Mudra. You have now activated Pingala Nadi. Then hold the breath while closing both nostrils and applying the Bandhas. Release the Bandhas, keep the right nostril closed with your thumb and exhale through the left.

U J J A Y I

51

CLOSING THE MOUTH, SLOWLY INHALE THROUGH BOTH NOSTRILS SO THAT IT RESONATES FROM THE THROAT TO THE CHEST.

52

DO KUMBHAKA AS BEFORE AND EXHALE THROUGH THE LEFT NOSTRIL. THIS REMOVES PHLEGM FROM THE THROAT AND IMPROVES DIGESTION.

53

THIS KUMBHAKA IS CALLED UJJAYI AND CAN BE DONE WHILE STANDING, SITTING OR WALKING. IT REMOVES DROPSY AND DISEASES OF THE NADIS AND DHATUS.

Inhale deeply through both nostrils, filling the lungs completely, apply the Bandhas and retain the breath. Release the Bandhas and exhale through the left nostril. When you practice Ujjayi, rasp the air through the nostrils, partially closing off the glottis. Suryabheda and Ujjayi both heat the body, and therefore exhalation is done through the left nostril, the path of the Ida Nadi, which has a cooling effect.

Nowadays it is advised to do Ujjayi throughout your Asana practice. When done in this way, it is a variation of Ujjayi Pranayama. You breathe deeply through the nose, rasping the air against the glottis without applying Kumbhaka. But when performed as a Kumbhaka, it should be practiced as described in this Sloka.

Ujjayi tones the nervous and digestive systems and removes excess phlegm, wind and bile. It Asana practice, it improves concentration and keeps the body energized

SITKARI

54

DRAW THE AIR THROUGH THE MOUTH MAKING THE SOUND "SEET" AND EXHALE THROUGH THE NOSE. ONE BECOMES A SECOND KAAMADEVA THROUGH THIS PRACTICE.

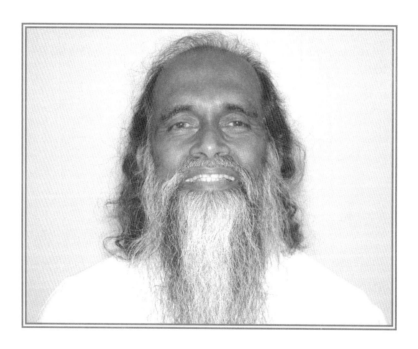

The practice of Sitkari, a cooling breath, is necessary as a counterbalance to Suryabheda and Ujjayi Pranayama, which are very heating. When you inhale through the mouth making the sound "seet," it is as if you are hissing as you press the tip of your tongue against the upper palate. It is believed that by practicing Sitkari, you become a second Kaamadeva, the god of love, and you attain a strong attractive aura.

55

**HE IS ADORED BY THE CIRCLE OF YOGINIS AND BECOMES THE CON-
TROLLER OF CREATION AND DISSOLUTION. HE IS NOT AFFLICTED
WITH HUNGER, THIRST, SLEEP OR LAZINESS.**

Through the practice of Sitkari, one is adored by the Circle of Yoginis, becomes
the controller of creation and dissolution, a god of love, free from hunger, thirst
sleep and laziness. How can breathing like that produce all these effects?

The reference to "Circle of Yoginis" and "controller of creation and dissolution"
refers to the creative aspect of the universe. A Yogini is the name for a female Yogi
and represents the feminine energies or the embodiment of Shakti, the Divine
mother, the cosmic creative force. A Yantra is a geometrical representation of
Shakti, in other words, the energy that represents the Divine aspect and an image
of cosmic wholeness. A Mantra is the sound or vibrational aspect of that specific
manifestation of God. For each Mantra, there is also a Yantra.

The Sri Yantra is one of the most well-known sacred Hindu Tantric symbols. It is
a Mandala, with 3 circles and 64 interlocking triangles within the innermost circle, representing the soul's evolution from the grossest to the subtlest state of consciousness. It is the representation of the Divine Mother in its totality or the fullness of the creative power, the Shakti. It is also the symbolic form of the sacred
sound of "Om" and represents Self-Realization, the merging of individual consciousness with the Supreme Consciousness.

The 64 interlacing triangles represent the 64 Yoginis, or in other words, the 64
aspects of Shakti. Within each individual, all of these 64 Yoginis are present. Even
though most of us are aware of only a few of these Indriyas, such as the eyes, the
ears, the nose and the mouth, this Divine energy is ever-present. According to the

Scriptures, there are 64 Indriyas, Gods, or Devas that are serving the individual as the different functionsin in the three bodies and five sheaths. We are endowed with the full power of creation, preservation and dissolution. Even though we are not conscious of it, it is happening all the time. The cells in the body are constantly created, preserved and destroyed. That power and all those Yoginis, as different manifestations of Shakti, are always within us.

As you proceed to the more subtle levels of consciousness, drawing your focus inward, you become aware of and experience those other Yoginis. That is when you are able to consciously gain control of the creative, preserving and dissolutive powers. It is through Yogic practice, not only specifically Sitkari, but any practice that leads to inner awareness, control and peacefulness of mind, that you reach the state where you are able to transcend limited awareness and experience the higher reality or Self, which is free from hunger, thirst, sleep, etc.

56
THROUGH THIS PRACTICE, THE BODY BECOMES PURE SATTWA AND HE IS REGARDED AS LORD OF THE YOGIS ON EARTH.

The three Gunas are Tamas, Rajas and Sattwa. Each of these forces is present in all individuals, although only one is dominating the personality at any one time. Tamas is characterized by laziness and dullness, which yields ignorance. Rajas is characterized by activity and passion, which yields pain. Sattwa is characterized by peacefulness and yields joy. Through the practices of Kumbhaka, Sattwa is enhanced. Sattwa is not really increased since it is already your nature. But as Tamas and Rajas within your personality are removed, Sattwa shines forth more and more. It is the polluting aspect of the other Gunas, Rajas and Tamas which, in effect, veils Sattwa. A Yogi who has reached the state of pure Sattwa is in a constant state of peace and is therefore always in awareness of his Higher Self.

Sitali

57

PROTRUDE THE TONGUE AND DRAW THE AIR IN. PRACTICE KUMBHA-KA AND EXHALE THROUGH THE NOSE.

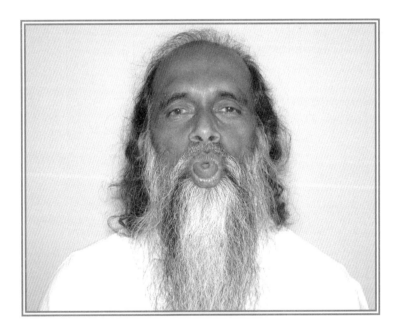

58

THIS KUMBHAKA IS CALLED SITALI AND CURES DISEASES LIKE GLAN-DULAR ENLARGEMENTS, DISORDERS OF SPLEEN AND BILE, AND COUN-TERACTS POISONS, HUNGER AND THIRST.

Sitali is the cooling breath. Breathing through the mouth in this manner will cool the mouth, throat and lungs, reduce high blood pressure and improve digestion. When you perform Sitali, curl your tongue as you stick it out and sip in the air. Then retain the breath and exhale through the nose.

BHASTRIKA

59

IN PADMASANA, WHERE BOTH FEET ARE CROSSED AND PLACED ON
OPPOSITE THIGHS, ALL SINS ARE DESTROYED.

60

BEING STABLE IN PADMASANA, KEEPING THE NECK AND BODY HELD
ERECT, EXHALE FORCEFULLY THROUGH THE NOSE.

61

THEN AGAIN THE AIR SHOULD BE INHALED FORCEFULLY SO THAT THE
RESOUNDING IS FELT FROM THE HEART, THROAT AND UP TO THE CRA-
NIUM.

62

THE YOGI SHOULD EXHALE AND INHALE IN THE ABOVE MANNER
AGAIN AND AGAIN WITH SPEED AND AWARENESS JUST AS A BLACK-
SMITH PUMPS HIS BELLOWS.

63

WHEN TIREDNESS IS FELT, INHALE DEEPLY THROUGH THE RIGHT NOS-
TRIL.

64

WHEN THE LUNGS ARE COMPLETELY FULL, RETAIN THE BREATH BY
HOLDING THE NOSTRILS WITH THE THUMB AND RING FINGER OF THE
RIGHT HAND.

65

HAVING RETAINED THE BREATH TO CAPACITY, EXHALE THROUGH THE
LEFT NOSTRIL. THIS INCREASES THE HEAT IN THE BODY, AND IMBAL-
ANCES OF WIND, BILE AND MUCUS ARE REMOVED.

Bhastrika means "bellows." It is comparable to Kapalabhati, except that the emphasis is also on the inhalation. As you continue to become more and more proficient in this practice, you will be using the entire breathing mechanism and all the muscles that are involved in breathing, just like a bellows pumping. Start with ten and gradually increase the pumps. Inhale through the right nostril. Apply Mula Bandha and Jalandhara Bandha as you retain the breath. Release the Bandhas and exhale through the left nostril as you do Udiyana Bandha and hold the breath for awhile externally. Bhastrika also heats the body and it is very good for the nervous and circulatory systems.

**66
IT AWAKENS KUNDALINI QUICKLY AND IS PLEASANT AND BENEFICIAL
TO REMOVE IMPURITIES AND EXCESS MUCUS BLOCKING THE
ENTRANCE OF BRAHMA NADI.**

**67
THIS KUMBHAKA IS CALLED BHASTRIKA AND SHOULD BE PRACTICED
REGULARLY FOR IT OPENS THE THREE GRANTHIS.**

The Granthis are the three safety valves or knots that God has created so that this Divine energy would not be prematurely awakened and create a short circuit within you. They can be found within the Sushumna Nadi. The Brahma Granthi is in the Muladhara Chakra, the Vishnu Granthi is in the Anahata Chakra and the Rudra Granthi is in the Ajna Chakra. Safety knots like that are not only present in each individual, they are inherent in every atom of creation. Without them, we would be having atomic explosions all the time. This planet would be the sun again.

The Granthis must be pierced and Bhastrika is a very powerful form of Pranayama which accomplishes this. You have to be careful with it because you do not want to short circuit the system. You have to reach a certain level of purity before you can start practicing Bhastrika. Prior to practicing any of the Kumbhakas, the Nadis have to be purified. And this does not simply mean having a nice flexible body. The mind has to be scrutinized very honestly. An aspirant has to scan his mind for selfishness, greed, anger, hatred, lust, jealousy, envy and fear. He must work sincerely to overcome these negative qualities.

If you cannot cope with emotional problems, imagine the state you would be in if that negative energy is increased many times through the effect of Pranayama! If your love and compassion increase by a hundred times, of course you will be ever so happy. But if your selfishness, greed, anger, hatred, lust, jealousy, envy and fear increase by a hundred times, no lunatic asylum will be able to take care of you. That is why it is so important to have a Guru to guide you safely through this spiritual awakening. It is a systematic and step-by-step process.

BHRAMARI

68

INHALE QUICKLY MAKING A REVERBERATING SOUND OF A MALE BEE AND EXHALE SLOWLY MAKING THE SOUND OF A FEMALE BEE. THIS IS BHRAMARI WHICH FILLS THE MIND OF THE YOGI WITH BLISS.

Bhramari is known as the humming breath and is a very good exercise to obtain a clear singing voice and to internalize the mind. In the practice of Bhramari, you inhale through both nostrils while partially closing the glottis, which creates a reverberating sound resembling a male bee. During the exhalation plug your ears with your index finger, make a humming sound like a female bee and feel the vibration in the cranium.

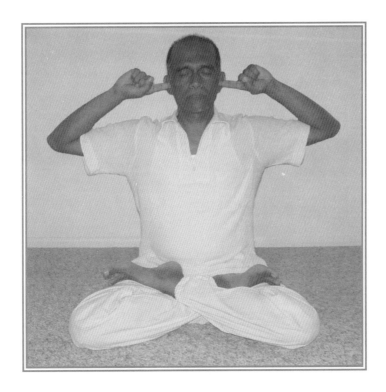

MURCHHA

69

INHALE DEEPLY AND APPLY JALANDHARA BANDHA FIRMLY THEN EXHALE SLOWLY. THIS IS CALLED MURCHHA AND CAUSES THE MIND TO SWOON AND GIVE PLEASURE.

The purpose of Murchha is to expand your consciousness and to store Prana. "Murchha" actually means "to swoon." But that does not mean that you should feel lightheaded when you do it. If that is the case, you should stop. You need to have reached a high degree of purification and a certain degree of control over the Prana to practice Murchha properly. It should also be done under the guidance of a Guru.

If done properly, Murchha will purge the mind of extraneous thoughts. It will also withdraw the mind from sensual pleasures and the external world, thereby bringing the awareness inward to experience a deeper inner peace. You will enter a relaxed state of being, leaving behind your anxiety and mental tensions.

PLAVINI

70

BY SWALLOWING AIR AND FILLING THE STOMACH COMPLETELY, THE YOGI CAN FLOAT ON THE DEEPEST WATER LIKE A LOTUS. THIS IS PLAVINI.

Continuously swallow air and fill up the belly, which will enable you to float in the water like a lotus leaf just for fun! However, if you do not have control and gulp in all that air, you might experience excruciating pain, especially if you do not know how to regurgitate it back. Today, people have flotation tanks to help induce a state of calmness. In those days, they were able to just lie in the water and float to induce the state of relaxation and peace.

71

PRANAYAMA IS A PROCESS OF INHALATION (RECHAKA), EXHALATION (PURAKA) AND RETENTION (KUMBHAKA). RETENTION (KUMBHAKA) IS OF TWO TYPES, VOLUNTARY (SAHITA) AND INVOLUNTARY (KEVALA).

Kumbhaka is the retention of breath. When the breath is retained consciously, it is called Sahita Kumbhaka. When the breath stops spontaneously, it is called Kevala Kumbhaka.

Prior to this, one must practice breathing exercises and purification of the Nadis: Abdominal Breathing, Full Yogic Breathing and Alternate Nostril Breathing. All these help to purify the Nadis. You will know when you have reached that state in your practice when both nostrils are open, your Asana practice is effortless and you can feel the Prana flowing.

72

SAHITA KUMBHAKA SHOULD BE PRACTICED UNTIL KEVALA KUMBHA-KA IS PERFECTED.

Before spontaneous suspension of the breath occurs, one should consciously practice Sahita Kumbhaka, retention of the breath, which will help to gain control of the Prana and the mind since they are inextricably intertwined. Sahita Kumbhaka can be done with Mantra repetition.

73

KEVALA KUMBHAKA IS WHEN THERE IS SUSPENSION OF BREATH WITH-OUT INHALATION OR EXHALATION.

Kevala Kumbhaka is suspension of breath without conscious effort. Kevala Kumbhaka occurs when Prana and mind cease moving.

74

THERE IS NOTHING IN THE THREE WORLDS THAT IS UNOBTAINABLE BY THE YOGI WHO HAS MASTED KEVALA KUMBHAKA AND CAN ENTER IT AT WILL.

Through the practice of Kumbhakas, the breath is retained with effort and becomes easier in time. Eventually the state is reached where the breath is suspended at will. This is Kevala Kumbhaka.

75

BY THE PRACTICE OF KUMBHAKAS, THE SUSHUMNA IS PURIFIED AND UNBLOCKED AND THE KUNDALINI SHAKTI IS AWAKENED AND SUCCESS IN HATHA YOGA TAKES PLACE.

76

THERE IS NO PERFECTION IN HATHA YOGA IF RAJA YOGA IS NOT REACHED AND NO SUCCESS IN RAJA YOGA WITHOUT HATHA YOGA. THEREFORE, PRACTICE UNTIL THE HIGHEST GOAL IS REACHED.

There is no perfection of Hatha Yoga unless Raja Yoga is attained. The term "Raja Yoga" here refers to a state that is reached, not a system of practice. Raja Yoga is the highest state, where one experiences his Oneness with the Supreme Conciousness. It is the result of total one-pointedness of mind. This total focus of mind can only be maintained when the body has been fully prepared. You cannot experience the state of Raja Yoga unless the body has been prepared step-by-step. You must go through the purification process. This systematic practice of Hatha Yoga should not stop until it culminates in the state of perfection called Raja Yoga.

77

THROUGH KUMBHAKA, THE PRANA IS CONTROLLED, WHICH FREES THE MIND OF MODIFICATIONS. THUS, ONE ACHIEVES THE STATE OF RAJA YOGA, SUPREME UNION.

A purified and concentrated mind reflects the Self or God, in the same way as a lake reflects the sun when there are no ripples on the surface.

Contrary to that state, the average mind is a bundle of thoughts that, like ripples, distort the perception of the reality that the individual self is one with the Supreme Self. Those ripples are called Vrittis or mental modifications. Thus, the cessation of the Vrittis is the goal of Yoga. This is achieved through the practice of Kumbhaka which gives control of Prana. When Prana is controlled, the agitation of the mind ceases, and then one experiences his identity with the Supreme Self. This is the state of perfection or Raja Yoga.

78

THE BODY BECOMES LEAN AND HEALTHY, THE EYES ARE CLEAR, THE FACE GLOWS WITH DELIGHT AND IS TRANQUIL, THE ANAHATA NADA MANIFESTS, THE BINDU IS UNDER CONTROL AND THE APPETITE INCREASES. THESE ARE SIGNS THAT THE NADIS ARE PURIFIED AND SUCCESS IN HATHA YOGA IS APROACHING.

These are indications of success in the practice of Hatha Yoga and a summary of all the effects you will experience as you move towards that state of perfection. If one is practicing Hatha Yoga properly, one will experience leanness of the body. A person who is overweight, clearly has not been practicing Hatha Yoga. That does not mean that he is not a Yogi because he might practice Bhakti Yoga or Karma Yoga, for instance. There are certain effects of each type of practice. But if you are observing all the rules of Hatha Yoga step-by-step, your body will rid itself of excess fat and become lean and healthy.

When the mind is calm and centered, it is able to go beyond audible sounds and mental conceptions, thus transcending the Vaikhari and Madhyama states of vibration. Vaikhari is the gross level where vibrations can be perceived as audible sound in the form of music, languages, etc. In the Madhyama state, vibration reaches the mental level and can be related to in the form of a universal concept. The Pashyanti state is more subtle. This is a transcendental state where vibration cannot be conceived by the mind. When the mind enters the Pashyanti state, the Anahata sound is heard. "Anahata" means "non-struck." Unlike the sounds that we hear on the Vaikhari level, it is not produced by two things being struck, but by the vibration of Akasha, ether.

There are different frequencies to the Anahata sound and they are related to the degree of purity of the Nadis, the time and degree of concentration and the intensity of the flow of Prana. In this state, you will become very aware of the subtle vibrations of the Prana. Eventually, the mind absorbed in the Anahata sound, will enter into the Para state, the most subtle level of vibration, where God is experienced directly as Nadam, pure vibration referred to as "Om."

Most people have no control of Bindu, which is the semen or ova. Whenever mating season comes for most species, the sexual urge becomes so strong that they would give their life to release it. Some animals mate once a year, whereas for some human beings, every night is mating season. Such excessive indulgence in sexual activity dissipates one's energy and scatters the mind.

Through the practice of Hatha Yoga, one can gain control over this sexual energy. After eating, food is broken down in the different Dhatus or tissues and the essence of it is used to build Shukra Dhatu, which is the reproductive cells. According to Master Sivananda, people naturally want to express that energy every thirteen to fourteen days. Once that energy is expressed, new Shukra Dhatu starts to build up and the cycle commences again. For Yogis however, the sexual energy does not have to culminate in that expression because Shukra Dhatu can be transmuted into Ojas Shakti, which is mental energy, and then into Tejas and Prana. This is how you gain control over the sexual energy. For the Yogi, control does not mean how long one can have sex. It means that he can transmute this lower form of energy into higher mental energy.

This transmutation process takes place through all kinds of Sadhana, not only Hatha Yoga techniques. It can also be achieved through Nada Yoga (music), Bhakti Yoga, prayers, reading good books and right association because sex impulses are triggered mainly by your mind and by association. Through the practice of Asana, Pranayama and other forms of Sadhana, the energy can be sublimated in every meaningful activity. It is mostly by habit that people desire sex because their thoughts are immersed in it. Wherever your thoughts are, that is where you send and concentrate your energy. As a result of that focus, the energy wants to express itself. Energy goes where attention flows. That is why in Tantric Yoga, misinformed people tend to concentrate on the lower Chakras like the Muladhara, Swadisthana and Manipura Chakras. People of wisdom, however, learn to focus on the Ajna Chakra which is the seat of consciousness. By focusing there, the energy is sublimated naturally without realizing it.

Chapter Three

MUDRAS

1

JUST AS THE LORD OF THE SERPENTS, SHESHANAGA, IS THE SUPPORT OF THE EARTH WITH ITS MOUNTAINS AND FORESTS, SO IS KUNDALINI THE SUPPORT OF ALL YOGA PRACTICES.

In this Sloka, reference to "Sheshanaga" means the cosmic Prana. Just as the support of the earth, mountains and forests is Sheshanaga, which is really cosmic Prana since life in any form cannot exist without Prana, similarly, Kundalini is the support of all Yogic practices. Kundalini is the power in the form of a coiled serpent that resides in the Muladhara Chakra. If you read the Puranas, there is an explanation of how Sheshanaga is related to the earth, the equator, the axis, etc.

2

BY THE GRACE OF THE GURU, THE SLEEPING KUNDALINI IS AWAKENED AND THE CHAKRAS AND GRANTHIS ARE OPENED.

This means that without the instructions or guidance of the Guru, you will get lost in all kinds of superstition and delusion if you try to awaken Kundalini on your own. You can read books and engage in all sorts of practices on your own but in reality, your mind will just be fantasizing about what this means. As the Kundalini is awakened and starts to move through the Chakras, you will be entering unknown territory: emotional, physical, psychic and spiritual. Whereas if the Guru is instructing, showing and teaching you step-by-step what it means, you will be successful in moving Kundalini through each of the Chakras until it reaches its final destination, the Sahasrara Chakra, where it unites with the Supreme Consciousness.

You must first go through an intense purification process and it is the Guru who will decide when you are ready. So it is only through the grace of a Guru that you are practicing your discipline, awakening the Kundalini and channeling it in the right direction. Yoga means realization of your Oneness with the Supreme Consciousness, which can only take place when you go beyond this relative awareness. It is a step-by-step process. You need the help of a Guru to unite Apana and Prana, to open the Sushumna and to break the Granthis (knots). As stated in one of the Meera Bhajans, "Using the boat of Truth and the Guru as the navigator, I have no anxiety of crossing this ocean of worldliness."

3
THEN SUSHUMNA BECOMES THE PATHWAY FOR PRANA, MIND IS WITH-OUT MODIFICATIONS AND DEATH IS AVERTED.

Once Sushumna is purified, then Prana begins to flow through it and your mind will cease fluctuating. Then death is averted. What does it mean when they say "death is averted?" It means that you are now identifying with who you really are, the true Self. When most people talk about "death," they are just associating and identifying with the body and relative experience. Once there is no modification of the mind, then man abides in his real nature, in complete awareness of the Self. In that sense, there is no death. When you reach this state, you can change bodies as many times as you change clothes but you remain fully aware of your true Self, who you really are.

Ignorant people think that the phrase "death is averted" means that they will live forever in this body. But immortality is not of the body. It is going beyond body consciousness and body awareness. That can only happen when you experience that state of Unmani, one-pointedness, no mind, where there is no fluctuation of mind. And that is the goal of Yoga, "Yoga Chitta Vritti Nirodha." Yoga is the control of all the thought waves in the mind or the stilling of all mental modification. When this happens, man abides in his real nature. At all other times, he identifies with the thought waves in his mind.

> 4
>
> **SUSHUMNA, SHUNYA PADAVE, BRAHMARANDHRA, MAHA PATHA, SHAMSHAN, SHAMBHAVI AND MADHYA MARGA ARE ALL DIFFERENT NAMES FOR THE SAME.**

> 5
>
> **THEREFORE MUDRAS MUST BE PRACTICED PROPERLY TO AROUSE THE GODDESS KUNDALINI SLEEPING AT THE ENTRANCE OF BRAHMA'S DOOR.**

These Slokas clearly illustrate how the systematic practice of Hatha Yoga brings purification of the Nadis, culminating in the purification of the Sushumna Nadi. When Prana starts to flow through Sushumna, then there is steadiness of mind. At that point, the mind becomes very concentrated and focused. And then you are ready for the arousal of Kundalini.

So many people say, "I want to raise Kundalini." When people are struggling and doing all the advanced techniques of Pranayama with the expectation, stress and anxiety of wanting to raise Kundalini, they are defeating the whole process. Their mind is getting in the way. You have to go through the entire process of Asana and Pranayama, starting with Abdominal Breathing, Full Yogic Breath, Kapalbhati and Alternate Nostril Breathing. Become established in Sattwic diet, Yamas and

Niyamas, right living, right thinking and right attitude. Then you will be ready to raise Kundalini.

Hatha Yoga Pradipika is a whole, integrated step-by-step process about how to purify and refine the systems, not just the physical body but the senses, mind, intellect and ego. It guides you how to withdraw from the world, which means you reach the state where you are no longer pulled by the world. It is only then that your mind will be still and your Prana will start to flow through Sushumna. It is not just the techniques, even though all the Sadhana that you are doing is helping you to gain centeredness, withdrawal and purity of mind. In essence, that is what is meant by practicing properly.

Once the Nadis are purified, and Prana is flowing through the Sushumna, your mind will be in a state of complete focus and concentration. Then you can practice Mudras to arouse Kundalini Shakti.

NAMES OF MUDRAS

6

MAHA MUDRA, MAHA BANDHA, MAHA VEDHA, KHECHARI, UDDIYANA, MULA BANDHA, JALANDHARA BANDHA.

7

VIPAREETA KARANI, VAJROLI AND SHAKTI CHALANA ARE THE TEN MUDRAS THAT DESTROY OLD AGE AND DEATH.

You will find the terms "destroy old age and death" throughout the *Hatha Yoga Pradipika*. People superstitiously identify with this statement. It also continuously states that the body becomes young. This really means that you can maintain youthfulness and good health for a long time but it does not mean immortality of the body. Remember, if you are still obsessed with body, body, body, then you are not going to move beyond body consciousness to experience anything higher.

8

SHIVA TAUGHT THESE MUDRAS THAT BESTOW THE EIGHT MAHA SIDDHIS. THESE ARE HELD IN HIGH ESTEEM BY THE SIDDHAS AND ARE DIFFICULT EVEN FOR THE GODS TO ATTAIN.

The eight Maha Siddhis referred to here are: Anima, the ability to become as small as an atom; Laghima, the ability to become weightless and fly; Mahima, the ability to become as large as the universe; Garima, the ability to become heavy; Prapti, the ability to travel anywhere; Prakamya, the ability to stay under water and to maintain the body and youth; Vashitva, the ability to master the elements, to exercise control over all objects, whether animate or inanimate; and Ishatva, the ability to create and destroy at will. In his *Yoga Sutras,* Maharishi Patanjali cautions against seeking and using these powers because they are obstacles to liberation.

From the standpoint of the ego, they are desirable powers. But liberation is a desireless state. Therefore, the Yogi who is tempted with these powers and renounces them is more apt to reach Samadhi.

9
THESE MUST BE KEPT SECRET JUST LIKE A BOX OF TREASURE AND NOT TALKED ABOUT TO ANYONE JUST AS ONE WILL NOT DISCUSS WITH OTHERS HIS INTIMATE RELATIONSHIP WITH HIS WIFE.

The point here is that if you are talking about these things, then it is just the ego expressing itself and showing off to others. It is an indication that you have not reached that state of proper harmony and calmness of the mind. Therefore, this is another discipline for you: try not to impress people. There is simply no point in talking about these things to someone who has not even started Hatha Yoga practice. All you are doing is boasting and trying to show off what you know.

You would not talk about your intimate relationship with your wife or husband if you truly treasured them. If you did, you would only be boosting your own ego, trying to impress others. Similarly, you should not talk about these practices. Check the tendency of wanting to show off because it magnifies the ego. You may encounter all kinds of curiosity with your practice. People will inquire about the significance of different techniques but you will discover that the person really has no interest. They are just going to use it as a conversation piece. Sometimes, when you are talking to them about it, you can even see disgust in their faces. They are genuinely not interested. One person will be sleeping and another one will be anxiously waiting for you to finish. If they inquire casually and you see that they really have no interest, just tell them not to worry about it and leave it alone.

M A H A   M U D R A

10

PRESSING THE PERINEUM WITH THE LEFT HEEL, STRETCH THE RIGHT LEG FORWARD AND GRASP THE RIGHT FOOT WITH BOTH HANDS.

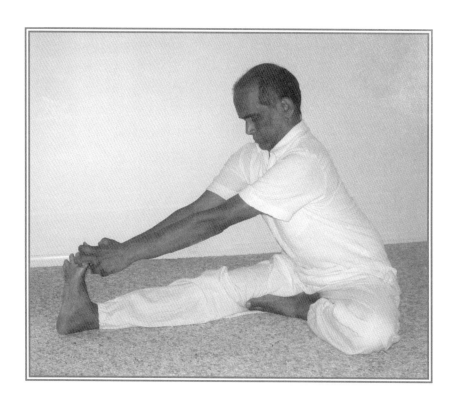

11

BY APPLYING JALANDHARA BANDHA AND RETAINING THE BREATH, KUNDALINI STRAIGHTENS JUST LIKE A SNAKE WHEN BEATEN WITH A STICK BECOMES STRAIGHT.

12

THEN IDA AND PINGALA BECOME INACTIVE AS THE SHAKTI ENTERS SUSHUMNA.

13

EXHALE SLOWLY AND GRADUALLY. THIS IS MAHA MUDRA AS DESCRIBED BY THE SIDDHAS.

14

BECAUSE THIS MUDRA DESTROYS THE WORST AFFLICTIONS AND EVEN DEATH, IT IS CALLED MAHA MUDRA.

15

REPEAT THIS PRACTICE ON THE OTHER SIDE. DISCONTINUE THE PRACTICE ONLY WHEN EQUAL NUMBER OF ROUNDS ARE PRACTICED ON BOTH SIDES.

16

FOR THE PRACTITIONER OF MAHA MUDRA THERE IS NOTHING THAT IS WHOLESOME OR UNWHOLESOME. ANY FOOD CAN BE CONSUMED, EVEN THE DEADLIEST POISON, AND IT WILL BE DIGESTED AND CONVERTED INTO NOURISHMENT.

17

ALL DISEASES LIKE CONSTIPATION, CONSUMPTION, INDIGESTION, LEPROSY, ETC. ARE REMOVED THROUGH THE PRACTICE OF MAHA MUDRA.

18

THUS MAHA MUDRA HAS BEEN EXPLAINED AS THE BESTOWER OF GREAT SIDDHIS. IT MUST BE KEPT SECRET AND IS NOT TO BE GIVEN TO JUST ANYONE.

Technique:

It is very simple. Press the perineum with the left heel. Stretch the right foot forward and grasp the right foot with the hands. Inhale deeply and apply Jalandhara Bandha and hold it for as long as you can. Exhale slowly and gradually. This is Maha Mudra.

These Mudras are very simple but people should not start doing them immediately. When you reach the state where the Sushumna and other Nadis are purified, the moment you start doing that Mudra, you feel the Kundalini straightening.

The Sloka states that it should be kept secret and it should not be given to just anyone. What will happen if you give it to anyone? After all, everyone wants advanced techniques. It only makes sense to someone who has reached that point in his practice. You can learn all the advanced techniques, practice Mudras all day and it will not make any difference. The only thing that will happen is that you will get a stiff neck or you will feel dizzy. It is not just something you do but rather the state that you reach. When you reach the state where the mind becomes so focused, you will experience the things described in these Slokas.

If you practice Maha Mudra, you can drink poison and eat anything you want, without it affecting you. You can simply convert it. It is not just the technique. But rather a state of consciousness that you reach. The story of Princes Meera illustrates this point. Princess Meera was an Indian princess and devotee of Krishna. When the prince's family became dissatisfied with her behavior because she was constantly associating with Yogis, Saints and devotees, singing and dancing in expression of her devotion for Lord Krishna, they tried to poison her with arsenic dissolved in milk. Meera did not practice Maha Mudra or anything like that. Yet when she drank the deadliest poison, it turned to nectar. It was because of her state of consciousness. All the techniques and disciplines explained here are designed to lead you step-by-step to elevate your consciousness to such a high state.

Some people will ignorantly interpret these Slokas to mean that Maha Mudra is a cure for poison. If that were the case, then they would be able to open a poison clinic and prescribe Maha Mudra. This is just silliness. That is why people relate to Yoga as therapy. It is a misuse or misrepresentation of the essence of Yoga. People advertise and make thousands of videos: Yoga for conception, Yoga for constipation, Yoga for asthma, Yoga for cats and dogs, etc. This is distorting the practice of Yoga.

M A H A   B A N D H A

19
PRESS THE LEFT HEEL IN THE PERINEUM AND PLACE THE RIGHT FOOT ON THE LEFT THIGH.

20
INHALE DEEPLY AND APPLY JALANDHARA AND MULA BANDHA. KEEP THE ATTENTION AND GAZE ON AJNA CHAKRA.

21
RETAIN THE BREATH FOR AS LONG AS POSSIBLE THEN EXHALE SLOWLY. REPEAT THIS PRACTICE ON THE OTHER SIDE.

22
SOME MASTERS ARE OF THE OPINION THAT JALANDHARA BANDHA IS NOT NECESSARY. THAT IT IS SUFFICIENT TO KEEP THE TONGUE AGAINST THE FRONT TEETH.

23
THIS MAHA BANDHA STOPS THE UPWARD MOVEMENT OF PRANA IN THE NADIS AND BESTOWS GREAT SIDDHIS.

24

MAHA BANDHA UNITES THE NADIS IN THE AJNA CHAKRA AND ENABLES THE MIND TO REACH THE SACRED SEAT OF SHIVA, KEDARA, THUS FREEING ONE FROM THE BONDS OF DEATH.

25

JUST AS THE CHARM AND BEAUTY OF A WIFE SERVE NO PURPOSE IN THE ABSENCE OF HER HUSBAND SO IS MAHA MUDRA AND MAHA BANDHA USELESS WITHOUT MAHA VEDHA MUDRA.

These three, Maha Mudra, Maha Bandha and Maha Vedha, are meant to be done together in order to awaken Kundalini Shakti and make her rise up the Sushumna. That is the purpose of awakening the Kundalini: so that she can move upward to unite with her Lord, Shiva.

MAHA VEDHA MUDRA

26

WHILE IN MAHA BANDHA, INHALE AND WITH A CONCENTRATED MIND, STOP THE MOVEMENT OF PRANA BY APPLYING JALANDHARA BANDHA.

27

PLACE THE PALMS ON THE GROUND, PUSH THE BODY UP AND GENTLY STRIKE THE BUTTOCKS ON THE GROUND BY BOUNCING UP AND DOWN. THIS CAUSES THE PRANA TO LEAVE THE TWO NADIS, IDA AND PINGALA, AND ENTER THE MIDDLE SUSHUMNA.

28

THIS UNION OF IDA AND PINGALA IN SUSHUMNA LEADS TO IMMORTALITY. A DEATHLIKE STATE IS EXPERIENCED, THEN EXHALE THE BREATH.

29

THIS MAHA VEDHA THAT GIVES GREAT SIDDHIS IS PRACTICED BY THE BEST YOGIS AND PREVENTS WRINKLES, GREY HAIR AND THE TREMBLING OF OLD AGE.

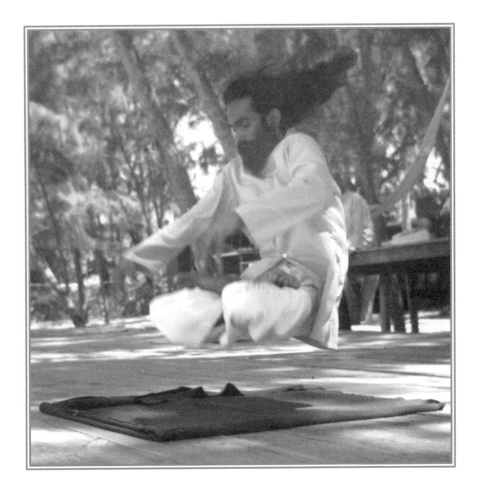

Sit in Padmasana and do Bhastrika Pranayama. During retention, place the palms on the floor and pushing the body up, bounce the buttocks on the floor several times. As is stated in the Sloka, this causes the Prana to leave Ida and Pingala and enter Sushumna. The body becomes charged with Prana. Kundalini is aroused and one experienccs a state of lightness of the body which makes it possible to jump higher and higher.

If you already have gray hair, etc, the point of Sloka 29 is that you can still slow down the aging process.

30
THESE THREE ARE THE GREAT SECRETS THAT DESTROY OLD AGE, DEATH, INCREASE DIGESTION AND BESTOW SIDDHIS LIKE ANIMA, ETC.

Here again youth is emphasized. All these practices will bestow health, slow down the aging process and bestow Maha Siddhis.

31
WITH PROPER INSTRUCTIONS, THEY SHOULD BE PRACTICED CAREFULLY EIGHT TIMES DAILY AT THREE HOUR INTERVALS. THEY BESTOW VIRTUES AND DESTROY VICES.

These instructions are not meant for just anybody. They are for the person who retires in his hermitage and is involved in practice 24 hours a day, with his mind completely withdrawn from the world. He has no anxieties or worries. It is meant for the person who has fulfilled his worldly obligations and duties.

KHECHARI MUDRA

32
TURN THE TONGUE BACKWARDS INTO THE CAVITY OF THE CRANIUM AND FIX THE GAZE ON AJNA CHAKRA. THIS IS KHECHARI MUDRA.

33
THIS IS ACHIEVED BY GRADUALLY CUTTING THE FRENUM LINGUE, EXERCISING AND MILKING THE TONGUE TO LENGTHEN IT SO THAT IT TOUCHES THE EYEBROW CENTER.

If you see someone do that, you would probably laugh. That is why people think Yogis are crazy. They cannot see beyond the physical aspect of what is happening. Why should this practice seem so bizarre when people pierce their tongues? If they can go through that kind of discipline, then cutting the frenum lingue should not disturb them. But even if they performed Khechari as instructed here, the benefits of Khechari will not be realized if they are not at the necessary level of consciousness yet.

34
WITH A SHARP STERILE BLADE, CUT THE FRENUM A HAIR'S BREADTH EACH TIME.

35
THEN RUB IN A MIXTURE OF POWDERED ROCK SALT AND TURMERIC. AFTER SEVEN DAYS CUT A HAIR'S BREADTH AGAIN.

Today, there are surgeons who can cut the whole frenum linguae all at once so that you do not have to go through this torture of cutting so many times. But the reason you cut only a hair's breadth each time is to develop discipline of the mind. This practice leads to withdrawal of the mind. Therefore, this practice of cutting the frenum lingue is really for discipline, not just to get the tongue out so that it touches the eyebrow center.

Turmeric is an antiseptic and that is why you are instructed to rub it on the area where the incision is made.

36
DO THIS REGULARLY FOR ABOUT SIX MONTHS UNTIL THE MEMBRANE IS COMPLETELY SEVERED.

This is a form of Tapas so that you develop the necessary discipline. It is simply another process that you undergo in the practice of Yoga.

37
TURN THE TONGUE BACK IN THE PATH OF THE THREE. THIS IS KHECHARI MUDRA AND IS CALLED VYOMACHAKRA.

The path of the three means the Ida, Pingala and Sushumna.

38
THE YOGI WHO REMAINS IN KHECHARI MUDRA EVEN FOR HALF A SECOND IS FREED FROM POISON, DISEASE, OLD AGE AND DEATH.

At that point in Khechari, when the mind completely stops, even for a fraction of a second, you experience your real nature. Vedanta philosophy uses the imagery of a rope and a snake to illustrate this. In twilight, a man treads upon a rope and, mistaking it for a poisonous snake, he jumps in fear. Later he realizes that the snake was nothing but a rope and his fear vanishes. When you mistake the rope for a snake, you scream in agony. How much of the rope do you need to see in order to know it is not a snake? You only need to see a strand to know it is a rope. Then you have no more fear. The moment you experience a glimpse of your true nature, who you really are, the infinite Self, you are free from death, old age and disease. This means that you are not identifying with the body anymore. All you need is a glimpse, a fraction of a second. Quite likely, for people who have reached that state of consciousness, things such as disease and poison will not affect the body because the body is an extension of the mind, which has become purified.

39
THE YOGI WHO MASTERS KHECHARI IS NOT AFFLICTED BY DISEASE, DEATH, FATIGUE, SLEEP, HUNGER, THIRST OR UNCONSCIOUSNESS.

40

THE MASTER OF KHECHARI IS NOT SUBJECT TO DISEASE, KARMA OR DEATH.

The practice of Khechari can lead the Yogi to Samadhi, the state of Supreme Consciousness, beyond duality and Karma.

41

THE SIDDHAS NAMED THIS MUDRA KHECHARI BECAUSE THE MIND ENTERS VOID AS THE TONGUE ENTERS EMPTY SPACE.

42

IN KHECHARI THE SEMEN IS NOT DISCHARGED, EVEN IF THE YOGI IS EMBRACED BY A PASSIONATE WOMAN.

43

EVEN IF THE SEMEN ENTERS THE PENIS, IT IS SEIZED AND TAKEN UPWARDS BY YONI MUDRA.

44

WITH THE TONGUE TURNED UPWARDS, THE YOGI DRINKING THE NECTAR FLOWING FROM THE MOON CONQUERS PHYSICAL DEATH WITHIN FIFTEEN DAYS.

45

THE YOGI WHO DRINKS THE NECTAR DAILY IS NOT POISONED EVEN IF HE IS BITTEN BY THE KING OF SNAKES.

46

JUST AS FIRE DOES NOT LEAVE WHILE THERE IS FUEL AND THE FLAME DOES NOT LEAVE THE WICK THAT IS SOAKED IN OIL, SO THE SOUL DOES NOT LEAVE THE BODY THAT IS FULL OF THE NECTAR FLOWING FROM THE MOON.

47

HE IS CONSIDERED TO BE OF HIGH LINEAGE WHO EATS THE FLESH OF COW AND DRINKS THE IMMORTAL LIQUOR DAILY. OTHERS ARE A DISGRACE TO THEIR LINEAGE.

48

HERE, COW MEANS TONGUE AND WHEN IT ENTERS THE UPPER PALATE THIS MEANS EATING THE FLESH OF COW. THIS DESTROYS GREAT SINS.

49

IMMORTAL LIQUOR IS THE NECTAR FLOWING FROM THE MOON. WHEN THE TONGUE IS INSERTED IN THE CAVITY, HEAT IS PRODUCED WHICH CAUSES THE NECTAR TO FLOW.

50

WHEN THE TIP OF THE TONGUE CONSTANTLY TOUCHES THE CAVITY, THE NECTAR THAT FLOWS HAS A SALTISH, PUNGENT, BITTER AND SOUR TASTE. IT IS OF THE CONSISTENCY OF MILK, HONEY AND GHEE. DISEASE, OLD AGE, DEATH AND ATTACK FROM DEADLY WEAPONS ARE WARDED OFF. THE YOGI ATTAINS THE EIGHT SIDDHIS, IMMORTALITY AND ATTRACTS WOMEN OF PERFECTION.

51

WITH THE TONGUE IN THE CAVITY AND THE HEAD TURNED UPWARD, THE NECTAR FLOWS INTO THE VISHUDDI CHAKRA. THUS, DRINKING THE STREAM OF NECTAR AND MEDITATING ON THE SUPREME SHAKTI, THE YOGI IS FREED FROM DISEASE AND LIVES A LONG LIFE WITH A BODY AS BEAUTIFUL AND SOFT AS A LOTUS FLOWER.

52

THE CAUSE OF DEATH IS WHEN THE NECTAR THAT FLOWS FROM MERU, THE SOURCE OF THE NADIS, IS CONSUMED BY THE FIRE. THE WISE WHO KNOW THIS, PRACTICE KHECHARI, OTHERWISE PERFECTION OF THE BODY IS NOT ATTAINED.

53

IN THAT CAVITY, WHICH IS THE SOURCE OF KNOWLEDGE, THE FIVE NADIS CONVERGE. IN THAT VOID KHECHARI MUDRA SHOULD BE ESTABLISHED.

54

THERE IS ONLY ONE SEED OF CREATION; ONE MUDRA, KHECHARI; ONE GOD WHO IS INDEPENDENT OF EVERYTHING; AND ONE STATE, MANONMANI.

When these Slokas talk about the "nectar flowing from the moon" and the "nectar of immortality," they are referring to the nectar of immortality flowing from the Bindu Visarga, which is the psychic center at the upper portion of the cranial cavity. These practices are very mystical and cannot be understood without the guidance and instructions of a Guru.

According to the process as described here, the nectar of immortality supposedly flows continously from the center of the Bindu Visarga, where the moon resides, and is consumed by the fire, the sun located at the solar plexus. Thus one experiences old age and death. If one practice Khechari, this nectar will not be consumed by the fire and one will be freed from old age, disease, etc.

When the tongue is turned back in Khechari and touches the point where the three Nadis, the Ida, Pingala and Sushumna converge, then the Yogi is able to drink the nectar. In Khechari, the body becomes full with this nectar and one is bestowed with many wonderful gifts such as immortality, freedom from disease, control over reproductive fluids, youth, radiant health, and a beautiful soft body. That is the theory underlying the practice of Khechari.

Even though this is a mystical practice, there are physical benefits that manifest as a result of Khechari. While the Bindu, Ida, Pingala and Sushumna are all located in the astral body, they have their counterparts in the physical body as well. The Bindu corresponds to the pineal gland, which is situated in the cerebrum in the upper portion of the cranial cavity. The Nadis have their physical counterpart in the nervous system. In effect, the physical body is a manifestation of the astral body. On the physical level, the practice of Khechari affects the endocrine glands, hormonal production, reproductive secretions, brain functions, autonomic breathing, heart rate, emotions, hunger, thirst, the central nervous system and the body's biological clock and sleep patterns.

Sloka 48 states, "Here, cow means tongue and when it enters the upper palate this means eating the flesh of cow. This destroys great sins." The reference to eating the flesh of cow and drinking the immortal liquor has been greatly misconstrued, especially in Tantric Yoga. People think that feasting on meat, drinking wine and having sex constitutes Tantric Yoga. This is a blasphemy of the Scriptures and a reflection of their lower state of consciousness. Here, cow means tongue. To eat the cow, means to swallow the tongue. Drinking the liquor or wine is referring to the nectar flowing from the moon.

UDDIYANA BANDHA

55

UDDIYANA BANDHA IS SO NAMED BECAUSE BY THIS PRACTICE PRANA IS CONCENTRATED AT ONE POINT AND MADE TO FLOW THROUGH SUSHUMNA.

56

THE BANDHA BEING DESCRIBED IS CALLED UDDIYANA BECAUSE IT CAUSES THE GREAT BIRD PRANA TO FLY UPWARDS WITH EASE.

57

PULLING THE ABDOMEN IN AND THE NAVEL UP IS CALLED UDDIYANA BANDHA. THIS IS THE LION THAT CONQUERS THE ELEPHANT, DEATH.

58

REGULAR PRACTICE OF THIS BANDHA AS INSTRUCTED BY THE GURU MAKES EVEN AN OLD PERSON LOOK YOUNG.

59

THE ABDOMEN ABOVE AND BELOW THE NAVEL SHOULD BE DRAWN BACKWARDS TOWARDS THE SPINE. BY PRACTICING REGULARLY FOR SIX MONTHS, THE YOGI CONQUERS DEATH.

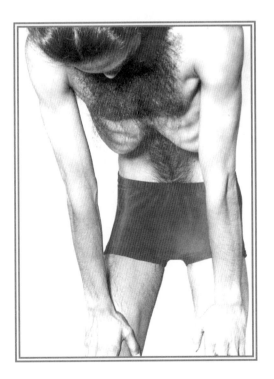
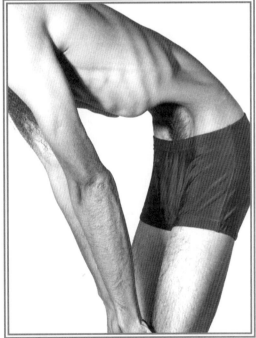

Again, you find that with all these Mudras, you are conquering death. How many times do you want to conquer death? The goal is to reach Samadhi, that state of Supreme Consciousness, liberation.

60

BY MASTERING UDDIYANA, LIBERATION COMES NATURALLY BECAUSE IT IS THE BEST OF ALL THE BANDHAS.

M U L A   B A N D H A

61

PRESS THE PERINEUM WITH THE HEEL. CONTRACT THE ANUS AND DRAW THE APANA UPWARDS. THIS IS MULA BANDHA.

While retaining the breath, contract the perineum muscles and then the abdominal muscle. This locks in the Apana, preventing it from escaping from the lower body and drawing it up so that it unites with Prana.

62

THE NATURAL TENDENCY OF APANA IS TO MOVE DOWNWARDS. BY CONTRACTING THE PERINEUM, IT IS FORCED TO GO UPWARDS. THIS IS CALLED MULA BANDHA.

Prana naturally moves up and Apana naturally moves down. With the practice of Mula Bandha, you help to reverse the flow of Apana.

63

PRESS THE ANUS FIRMLY WITH THE HEEL. FORCEFULLY AND REPEATEDLY CONTRACT THE PERENIUM UNTIL THE VITAL ENERGY RISES.

64

YOGA OR PERFECTION IS ATTAINED BY UNITING PRANA AND APANA, NADA AND BINDU THROUGH THE PRACTICE OF MULA BANDHA. THERE IS NO DOUBT ABOUT THIS.

65

BY REGULAR PRACTICE OF MULA BANDHA, URINE AND STOOL DECREASE AND EVEN THE OLD BECOME YOUNG.

66

WHEN APANA MOVES TO THE REGION OF FIRE, IT FANS THE FLAME.

67

WHEN APANA AND PRANA UNITE IN THIS FIRE CENTER, THE HEAT IN THE BODY INTENSIFIES.

68

DUE TO THIS INTENSE HEAT, THE SLEEPING KUNDALINI SHAKTI STRAIGHTENS AND HISSES JUST LIKE A SERPENT STRUCK BY A STICK.

69

THEN IT ENTERS THE BRAHMA NADI JUST LIKE A SERPENT ENTERS ITS HOLE. THEREFORE MULA BANDHA SHOULD BE PRACTICED EVERY DAY.

JALANDHARA BANDHA

70

CONTRACT THE THROAT BY BRINGING THE CHIN TOWARDS THE CHEST. THIS IS JALANDHARA BANDHA AND IT DESTROYS OLD AGE AND DEATH.

71

THIS JALANDHARA BANDHA CATCHES THE FLOW OF NECTAR IN THE THROAT AND DESTROYS ALL THROAT AILMENTS.

72

JALANDHARA BANDHA PREVENTS THE NECTAR FROM FALLING INTO THE FIRE AND FACILITATES THE STABILITY OF PRANA.

73

THROUGH JALANDHARA BANDHA THE TWO NADIS ARE RENDERED INACTIVE AND THE SIXTEEN ADHARAS IN THE MIDDLE CHAKRA ARE CONTROLLED.

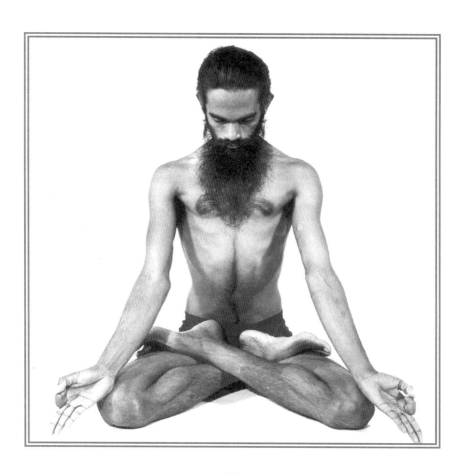

The Vishuddi Chakra is located in the Sushumna at the base of the throat. It has 16 petals or Adharas and is of a smoky purple color. The 16 Adharas referenced here are the 16 forms of Shakti or energy that emanate from this Chakra. Each petal is represented by a Bija Mantra: Am, Aam, Im, Eem, Um, Oum, Rim, Reem, Lrim, Lreem, Em, Aim, Om, Aum, Ah, Amh. Each Bija Mantra relates to various bodily functions, mental and psychic centers. The practice of Jalandhara Bandha prevents the nectar of the Bindu from flowing downward past the Vishuddi Chakra to be consumed by the fire in the solar plexus, the Manipura Chakra. This happens because Jalandhara Bandha effectively stops the flow of Shakti in the Ida and Pingala Nadis, thereby inducing it to flow through the Sushumna and collect in the Vishuddi Chakra.

74
THROUGH MULA BANDHA, UDDIYANA BANDHA AND JALANDHARA BANDHA, THE IDA AND PINGALA ARE CLOSED AND SUSHUMNA BECOMES ACTIVE.

75
BY THIS PRACTICE, THE BREATH IS SUSPENDED AND PRANA BECOMES STEADY. DEATH, OLD AGE AND SICKNESS ARE CONQUERED.

76
THESE THREE BANDHAS ARE REGARDED AS THE BEST OF ALL SAD-HANAS BY THE GREAT SIDDHAS. THEY RESULT IN SUCCESS IN THE HATHA YOGA PRACTICE.

77
WHILE THE NECTAR OF IMMORTALITY IS CONSTANTLY BEING CON-SUMED BY THE SUN, OLD AGE AND DEATH ARE INEVITABLE.

78
**THERE IS AN EFFECTIVE WAY TO PREVENT THE NECTAR FROM FALLING
INTO AND BEING CONSUMED BY THE SUN. THIS CAN ONLY BE
LEARNED FROM A GURU AND NOT FROM HUNDREDS OF SHASTRAS.**

These three Bandhas, Mula Bandha, Uddiyana Bandha and Jalandhara Bandha, should be practiced before you even reach this point. Incorporate these Bandhas in your practice of Anuloma Viloma for the purification of the Nadis, as instructed in chapter 2, verses 7-10.

Here again it is declared that Jalandhara Bandha is a method of preventing the nectar from being consumed by the sun. Since this objective is achieved in Jalandhara Bandha, you do not have to try and combine every technique mentioned in the *Hatha Yoga Pradipika*, such as cutting your tongue, Vajroli Mudra, Amaroli Mudra, etc. Any one of these will achieve the same objective.

VIPARITA KARANI MUDRA

79
**VIPARITA KARANI IS THE REVERSING PROCESS WHEREBY THE NAVEL
REGION IS ABOVE AND THE PALATE IS BELOW, THE SUN ABOVE AND
THE MOON BELOW. WHEN THIS INSTRUCTION IS GIVEN BY THE GURU,
IT LEADS TO SUCCESS.**

80
**THE DIGESTIVE FIRE INTENSIFIES THROUGH REGULAR PRACTICE.
THUS, THE PRACTITIONER SHOULD HAVE SUFFICIENT FOOD OR ELSE
HE WILL BE CONSUMED.**

This instruction is not meant for everybody and it certainly does not mean that you should eat everything in the refrigerator. It is meant for people who reach the stage where their digestive fire has increased so much that they need to eat sufficient food to sustain themselves and their energy.

81
WITH THE FEET ABOVE AND THE HEAD BELOW, ONE SHOULD REMAIN IN THIS POSITION FOR A SHORT TIME THE FIRST DAY AND GRADUAL-LY INCREASE THE DURATION EVERY DAY.

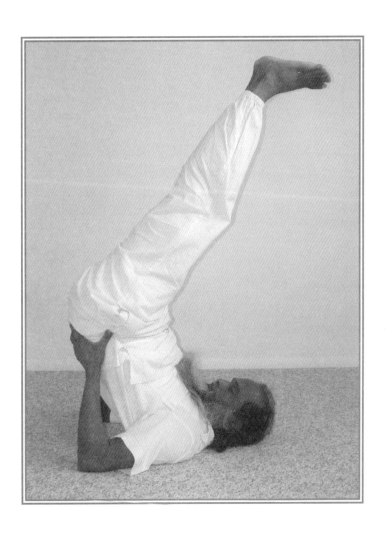

82

WRINKLES AND GREY HAIR DISAPPEAR AFTER SIX MONTHS OF PRACTICE. DEATH IS CONQUERED IF ONE PRACTICES REGULARLY FOR THREE HOURS DAILY.

Here again, the reversal of the aging process and the conquering of death in the inverted postures is mentioned. Why is it that people who are doing inverted postures cannot achieve these benefits? The secret is that when you practice headstand and shoulderstand, there is still effort in pushing up. But Viparita Karani is a more relaxed, natural form of this inverted posture. When you can remain in Viparita Karani or headstand without any effort at all, just like when you are standing on your feet naturally, then the body's mechanism has reached a state where there is no more awareness that you are inverted. That is when the nectar is not consumed but recirculated in the body. If there is effort involved, then the body knows that it is inverted and then the sun is still consuming the nectar.

Again you can see the indication that it is not just a physical thing. The mere fact that you are upside down does not mean that this nectar will not be consumed. It is a state of consciousness. Whether you are upside down or rightside up, the heart is still pumping blood and the body is still eliminating waste, absorbing nutrients, etc. The nature and intelligence of the body is to age and undergo the process of growing. But when that mechanism is tricked, as in Viparita Karani, the nectar does not go through the normal process of being consumed by the sun, which really means consumed by your effort. Then you remain in that state of youthfulness.

VAJROLI MUDRA

83

ONE WHO PRACTICES VAJROLI WELL BECOMES A SIDDHA EVEN IF HE DOES NOT FOLLOW THE RULES AND OBSERVANCES OF YOGA.

This may, at first, seem like a contradiction, but to be able to practice Vajroli well means that you have reached a level of discipline where you have control of the mind and the body. It is a very high state to attain. When you reach that level in your Sadhana, a state of control of mind, then there is no need for rules and discipline anymore. They cease to serve any purpose in your life. To the ordinary person, your actions and mode of life will be judged according to their own state of consciousness. You will be existing in a whole different state of consciousness, which will not conform to the rules and regulations that ordinary people need to follow for their evolution. Their relationship to sex and sensuality is quite different. It is one of indulgence that weakens the mind and senses.

84

FOR SUCCESS IN THIS PRACTICE, THERE ARE TWO THINGS THAT ARE DIFFICULT TO OBTAIN, ONE IS MILK AND THE OTHER IS A WOMAN WHO WILL ACT ACCORDING TO YOUR WILL.

The reference to milk must not be taken out of context. In those days, milk was quite difficult to obtain and was regarded as a precious thing. The Slokas are replete with references to things that apply only to that time period and in light of the existing circumstances. If you take them literally today, they will no longer make sense. This is a perfect example. Today, milk is not difficult to obtain in most countries although there are still certain places in the world where it is scarce. In this country, there are, of course, other things that are more difficult to obtain than milk.

The reference to finding a woman who will act according to your will means that if you are involved with somebody in the practice of Vajroli and your partner does not have the same level of consciousness or evolution, then you will be creating many problems for yourself, emotionally, socially and otherwise.

If you are married and your wife is practicing Sadhana, then she is the best person with whom to practice Vajroli Mudra. In that case, there are no social implications. But it is necessary for her to be practicing the same kind of Sadhana that you are practicing or else it is going to create problems and conflicts. Therefore, it is a very rare thing to find. For someone to practice Vajroli Mudra, the person must have a certain state of consciousness such that it is not another excuse to indulge in sexual activity and to call it Yoga. It should be done with detachment just like you do any other kind of Mudra or Kriya. Vajroli Mudra must be done within that context, with that kind of awareness and a high level of consciousness. If it is not practiced this way, it can really warp the mind of people and create all kinds of delusions and problems. There has to be that necessary clarity, maturity, state of evolution and consciousness. If you do not possess all these qualities, just leave it alone. You do not need to be involved in all these Mudras.

If you are a married spiritual aspirant and depending on your mode and station in life, your involvement in sex should be in moderation. It is just like eating; you eat moderately and avoid overeating. Instead of overindulgence, if you want to engage in sexual activity because of your partner, be involved in a loving, nice way. Do not fool yourself into thinking that you are doing Vajroli Mudra. These Slokas here are talking about techniques. Where is the question of love? There is no ingredient of love. It is just a pure act. When you are cleaning your tongue and doing Neti, you are not doing it with love. You are doing it as part of a process.

Even though there is love for the body and love for good health, we do not look upon it that way. Whereas in relationship with your spouse, it is an expression of love. Therefore, if one is involved in sex with that kind of awareness and consciousness, naturally it will help you to evolve and grow. Eventually, if you are involved in a systematic practice of Hatha Yoga, you will naturally reach the point where even this activity can be done in the manner as described.

85
BY GRADUALLY PRACTICING TO DRAW THE BINDU UP DURING EMISSION IN INTERCOURSE, THE MAN OR WOMAN WILL ACHIEVE SUCCESS IN VAJROLI.

86
GRADUALLY DRAW AIR THROUGH A PRESCRIBED TUBE INSERTED INTO THE URETHRA OF THE PENIS.

This practice is another exercise that you can do but you have to be very careful. In those days, they prescribed certain things, such as a metal tube made of gold, silver or copper. Today you can use a catheter lubricated with almond oil or ghee. You really must have great dispassion to want to perform this practice. In the same manner that people push a catheter through their nose, it takes a lot effort and perseverance to insert a tube into the urethra of the penis.

Why would someone want to do this? It is a very involved practice and very risky. After inserting the tube, you draw up air, then water, milk, honey, mercury, etc. I am of the opinion that you are either a very masochistic person or a very determined person to try this because you risk bladder infection, tearing the lining of the urethra and other kinds of infection. If you are really bent on this kind of pursuit, be very careful and confident that you are capable of doing it. While you are engaged in this process and you achieve that kind of success, then you will be able to draw up the Bindu.

Nevertheless, why would you want to emit the Bindu and then draw it back up again? You could see the paradox here. The mere fact that you are involved in sexual activity or sexual thoughts means that you are stirring up that energy. Why do you want to stir it up, release it, only to pull it up and conserve it? This is not practical and is a contradiction in itself. Instead, the Yogic way, the Sattwic way, is to really sublimate the energy. Sublimation means that you are involved in Sadhana, by thinking pure positive and divine thoughts, reading inspiring books, right association, observing proper diet, all of which will sublimate that energy naturally.

If you feast your mind on sexual activity by thinking about it, then you will arouse that energy. Even erection is not possible unless the mind comes down to that state and generates thoughts there. So it is like playing with fire. Why light a fire and then try to put it out? It is a dangerous practice. You will come to a point where you wonder how far this fire can burn as it continues to build and how many drapes it can burn before you try to extinguish it. In the process of putting out that fire, you create more problems and damage. Instead, take precautions not to light the fire in the first place.

My advice is that you just leave this practice alone and treat sex for what it is. If you are at that level of consciousness where you need to be involved in sex, be involved on a Sattwic level, a Dharmic level, where you are expressing love the way it should be done. That will help you to evolve, grow and develop love, compassion, warmth, closeness and similar qualities with somebody.

When someone reaches the state where he has control over senses and mind, where he can practice Vajroli and Amaroli, you may wonder why he would even feel the need to practice them. At that stage of evolution, it is merely to have some fun, like having ice cream. There is really no other relationship to it. Even the Gods want to have some fun from time to time and so they come down to earth. But if you want to have some fun, then you still have desires and thus, you are not fulfilled.

87
PRACTICE TO DRAW THE BINDU UP AS IT IS ABOUT TO FALL AND IF IT DOES, IT SHOULD BE DRAWN UP ALONG WITH THE WOMAN'S FLUID.

88
THE YOGI WHO CAN CONSERVE HIS BINDU CONQUERS DEATH. RELEASE OF BINDU LEADS TO DEATH WHILE ITS CONSERVATION PRE-SERVES LIFE.

The reference to conserving Bindu does not mean that you emit semen and then try to suck it back in again. If that were the case, it would be akin to eating food, vomiting it out and trying to swallow it back again. Why regurgitate it? Instead, why not try to assimilate the food? It does not make sense. It is a very unwise prac-tice. In the same way, this energy, namely the Bindu, the sexual energy, the Shukra Dhatu, can be assimilated and converted to Ojas Shakti, Tejas and Prana through your Sadhana.

The manufacture of the Bindu, Shukra Dhatu or sexual energy is a natural func-tion of the body and cannot be suppressed. Everything you ingest and imbibe through your senses is used to build this energy. This includes thoughts, the kind of books you read, what you hear, the kind of association you keep, etc. It is all food, which is used to build the different Dhatus, the different cells: plasma, muscle, fat, bone, marrow, nerves and reproductive tissue. The Shukra Dhatu, the sex cells, are like the essence of all the food that you ingest. In accordance with the normal, natural process, rhythm and cycle of the body, about every 13 days, your sexual impulses are aroused because it is nature's means of expressing itself for procreation and preservation of the species. But Yogis know this does not necessarily have to be the end product of the cycle of food. With their understanding and knowledge of the process, they can transmute the Shukra Dhatu not through suppression but through Sadhana and the art of right living. In fact, the reason why it is advised not to mix with the opposite sex in the very beginning of your Sadhana, is because you do not want to bring your mind to a state where it is stimulating and arousing sexual impulses. Instead, that energy is transmuted into Ojas Shakti, mental energy, into a brilliance, which you can see in someone's face. They will shine with Prana.

In the West here, many people are reducing this very sacred practice of Vajroli to the act of sex and then labeling it Tantra Yoga. They are creating numerous problems for themselves and are simply not aware of it because they are involved in delusion and ignorance. Rather than expressing or manifesting a state of brilliance by following what the Scriptures say, they are simply draining all their Prana. They are just manifesting the opposite results, shattering their senses and nervous system and scattering their mind. Many of them, even the ones who call themselves Masters, are often lost and involved in delusion. They drain their Prana and energy, focusing solely on how to hold off ejaculation as long as possible. In the process of doing that, they are shattering their nervous system and moving further and further away from the goal of Yoga. Open your eyes and see the truth. Use your discrimination. Do not fall prey and victim to propaganda and delusion.

CHAPTER 3 • MUDRAS

Sexual intercourse is a very superficial relationship to Vajroli Mudra. Tantric Yoga is a very involved practice, with all kinds of rituals to help you withdraw your mind and elevate your consciousness to a very high state. This sexual energy can be sublimated so that you do not have to deal with it in this way.

89
THE YOGI'S BODY HAS A PLEASANT SWEET SMELL WHEN THE BINDU IS PRESERVED. WHY SHOULD THERE BE FEAR OF DEATH WHEN THE BINDU IS PRESERVED?

90
MIND AND SEMEN SHOULD BE PROTECTED BECAUSE LIFE DEPENDS ON SEMEN AND SEMEN IS CONTROLLED BY MIND.

91
THE YOGI WHO IS ESTABLISHED IN THIS PRACTICE IS ABLE TO CON-SERVE BOTH HIS AND THE WOMAN'S BINDU BY DRAWING IT UP.

SAHAJOLI MUDRA

92
SAHAJOLI AND AMAROLI ARE VARIATIONS OF VAJROLI. THE ASHES OF BURNT COW MANURE ARE MIXED WITH WATER.

93
AFTER VAJROLI, SITTING IN THE STATE OF BLISS, THE YOGI AND YOGI-NI SHOULD SMEAR THE ASHES ON SPECIFIC PARTS OF THEIR BODIES.

Ashes signify renunciation. Thus, the act of smearing ashes on the body is a symbolic act of detachment and renunciation.

94

THIS IS SAHAJOLI AND THE YOGIS HAVE UNSHAKEABLE FAITH IN IT BECAUSE IT LEADS TO LIBERATION EVEN THOUGH IT IS MIXED WITH ENJOYMENT.

95

THE YOGI WHO IS ESTABLISHED IN VIRTUE, FREED FROM THE LOWER NATURE, WILL SUCCEED IN THIS YOGA WHEREAS OTHERS WILL FAIL.

The Sloka states clearly that it is only the Yogi who is established in virtue and freed from the lower nature who will succeed in this practice. Unless you reach that state of perfection or are established in the virtues of Yama and Niyama, where the mind is purified and you are freed from the lower nature of desires, lust, greed, etc., you will not succeed in Sahajoli. Instead, it will immerse you further and further into delusion and indulgence.

AMAROLI MUDRA

96

ONE OF THE PRACTICES OF THE KAPALIKA SECT IS AMAROLI, WHICH IS THE DRINKING OF THE MIDSTREAM OF THE URINE. THE FIRST AND LAST PARTS ARE LEFT BECAUSE THE FIRST PART CONTAINS TOO MUCH BILE AND THE LAST PART IS USELESS.

My feeling on this matter is, "To each his own." You do not have to do everything. This is urine therapy. If you are not sick, then why try to fix what is not broken? It is believed that urine contains many wonderful elements, nutrients, etc. The mere fact that it is being eliminated means that you have an excess in your body. Your body uses what it needs and gets rid of the rest. So why worry about it? If you feel depleted or sick, and you feel the need to use this kind of therapy, then go ahead. But you do not need to practice it every day and all the time. It is not going to enhance your spiritual awareness. In fact, you will become obsessed with this. I have encountered people who were supposedly experts on urine therapy. Every pore of their body oozed out urine. They reeked as if they were walking urine pots. That is because they regard every drop of urine as nectar and are not just drinking midstream as instructed by the Scriptures. Instead, they are drinking everything, which is a derangement.

97
THE YOGI WHO DRINKS AMARI THROUGH THE NOSE AND PRACTICES VAJROLI IS SAID TO BE PRACTICING AMAROLI.

98
THE YOGI GETS DIVINE SIGHT BY SMEARING THE UPPER PARTS OF THE BODY WITH A MIXTURE OF SEMEN AND ASHES OF BURNT COW MANURE.

99
A WOMAN IS A YOGINI WHO CAN PRACTICE VAJROLI BY DRAWING UP A MAN'S BINDU WHILE PRESERVING HERS.

100
IN THIS WAY, THERE IS NO WASTE AND NADA AND BINDU BECOME ONE IN THE BODY.

101
THUS PERFECTION IS ATTAINED WITH THE UNION OF NADA AND BINDU THROUGH THE PRACTICE OF VAJROLI.

102
THE YOGINI WHO IS SUCCESSFUL IN VAJROLI KNOWS THE PAST, PRESENT AND FUTURE AND BECOMES FIXED IN HIGHER CONSCIOUSNESS.

103
PERFECTION OF THE BODY IS AN EFFECT OF VAJROLI AND ALONG
WITH ENJOYMENT, LIBERATION CAN BE REACHED.

Through the Tantric practice of Vajroli, liberation can be attained. Here, the Sloka indicates that liberation can be reached through enjoyment and sensual experience. But this depends on how you relate to the senses. You will develop reverence for the senses once you know that they are Devatas or Gods serving you. Sexual energy is another manifestation of the Divine Shakti and when it is related to with this understanding and reverence, then the involvement in Vajroli, Amaroli and Sahajoli will lead to higher consciousness. If not, you will be using these practices as an excuse to abuse the senses, and thus displease the Devatas and outrage the Atman, and this is referred to as sin.

The goal is to awaken Kundalini Shakti at the Muladhara Chakra and to raise this Shakti up to the Sahasrara Chakra to unite with the Supreme Consciousness, to experience the true Reality. It is the union of opposite poles, of uniting energy, Shakti, with consciousness, Shiva.

104
KUTILINGI, KUNDALINI, SHAKTI, ISHVARI, KUNDALI AND ARUNDHATI
ARE ALL SYNONYMOUS TERMS.

105
JUST AS ONE OPENS A DOOR WITH A KEY, SO THE YOGI OPENS THE
DOOR TO LIBERATION WITH KUNDALINI.

106
KUNDALINI SLEEPS WITH HER MOUTH CLOSING THE DOOR THAT
LEADS TO THE ABODE OF BRAHMAN, THE PLACE BEYOND SORROW.

107
THE KNOWER OF YOGA KNOWS THAT KUNDALINI SHAKTI SLEEPING
ABOVE THE KANDA IS THE MEANS OF LIBERATION FOR THE YOGI AND
BONDAGE FOR THE IGNORANT.

The Yogi who understands clearly that his primary goal and purpose of life is to reach liberation, will use the power of Kundalini Shakti for that purpose. However, if liberation is not the primary objective, then the power will be used to exploit others, thus leading to further bondage.

108
KUNDALINI IS COILED LIKE A SNAKE. THE YOGI WHO MAKES THIS
SHAKTI MOVE WILL OBTAIN LIBERATION WITHOUT A DOUBT.

109
THE YOUNG WIDOW WHO IS PRACTICING TAPAS BETWEEN THE GANGA
AND YAMUNA MUST BE SEIZED FORCEFULLY IN ORDER TO REACH THE
HIGHEST ABODE OF VISHNU.

110
THE HOLY GANGA IS IDA, AND PINGALA IS THE HOLY RIVER YAMUNA.
IN THE MIDDLE IS THE YOUNG WIDOW KUNDALINI.

Here the Sloka draws an analogy that Kundalini is a widow because she is seperated from her beloved spouse, Shiva.

111
SEIZE THE TAIL OF THE SLEEPING SERPENT, KUNDALINI WHO WILL
AWAKEN AND START TO MOVE UPWARDS.

SHAKTI CHALANA MUDRA

112
INHALE THROUGH THE RIGHT NOSTRIL AND SEIZE THE SERPENT THROUGH KUMBHAKA AND ROTATE HER CONSTANTLY FOR ONE AND A HALF HOURS MORNING AND EVENING DAILY.

This is really a mental process. At this point in your practice, your mind should be one-pointed. When you are inhaling and holding your breath, your focus is on Kundalini Shakti, the serpent. To "rotate her" means that you are meditating and experiencing the movement of Kundalini Shakti. It is a continuous practice and you need to be involved in uninterrupted Sadhana. It is not something that happens all of a sudden. Suppose you want strong abdominal muscles. You do not develop those muscles after raising your legs one time. You must practice and have discipline to develop those muscles. It is the same with these practices and the Kumbhakas. It takes time and discipline. You must proceed step-by-step.

The same holds true for meditation and focusing your mind. For example, there are different types of meditations for the different Chakras, each of which has its own presiding deities. When you meditate on a Chakra, visualize the different petals and mentally repeat the appropriate Bija or sound for each petal, such as hum, yam, ram, tam, lam, etc. It is a very involved practice.

Therefore, when the Sloka instructs you to practice Shakti Chalana Mudra for one and a half hours morning and evening every day, that becomes your meditation. Your focus changes as you continue in your Sadhana. In the beginning, the focus is on purification of the Nadis. Next, you move onto Kumbhakas. Then you focus on Mudras and awakening the Kundalini Shakti.

Once you awaken it, you need to move into a different phase of Sadhana to direct the Kundalini Shakti. If it is not directed properly, it can lead to other problems. This is why the Sushumna must be purified and the Granthis pierced so that it travels through that central channel. These are the different step-by-step phases one must undergo.

113
THE KANDA IS TWELVE FINGERS ABOVE THE ANUS AND IS FOUR FINGERS WIDE. IT IS SOFT AND WHITE AND APPEARS LIKE A FOLDED CLOTH.

114
SITTING IN VAJRASANA, GRAB HOLD OF THE FEET NEAR THE ANKLES AND PRESS THE KANDA.

115
IN VAJRASANA, DO BHASTRIKA PRANAYAMA TO AROUSE KUNDALINI.

116
CONTRACT THE SUN IN MANIPURA AND MOVE KUNDALINI. EVEN IF ONE IS ON THE VERGE OF DEATH, THERE IS NO NEED TO FEAR.

117
FEARLESSLY MOVE KUNDALINI FOR ABOUT ONE AND A HALF HOURS AND DRAW HER UP SUSHUMNA A LITTLE.

118
BY THIS PRACTICE KUNDALINI LEAVES THE MOUTH OF SUSHUMNA. THIS ALLOWS PRANA TO FLOW UP SUSHUMNA NATURALLY.

119

BY MERELY MOVING KUNDALINI IN THIS WAY EVERY DAY, THE YOGI IS FREED FROM DISEASE.

120

THE YOGI WHO MOVES THE SHAKTI REGULARLY ENJOYS PERFECTION AND PLAYFULLY CONQUERS DEATH. WHAT MORE IS THERE TO SAY?

121

THE YOGI WHO DELIGHTS IN BRAHMACHARYA, EATS MODERATELY A SATTWIC DIET AND PRACTICES KUNDALINI AROUSAL, REACHES PERFECTION IN FORTY DAYS.

122

BHASTRIKA KUMBHAKA IS MOST EFFECTIVE IN ACTIVATING KUNDALINI. TO THE YOGI WHO PRACTICES IN THIS MANNER EVERYDAY, WHERE IS THE FEAR OF DEATH?

123

WHAT OTHER MEANS ARE THERE TO WASH AWAY THE IMPURITIES OF THE SEVENTY-TWO THOUSAND NADIS OTHER THAN THE PRACTICE OF KUNDALINI AROUSAL?

124

SUSHUMNA, THE MIDDLE NADI, BECOMES STRAIGHT BY THE REGULAR PRACTICE OF ASANA, PRANAYAMA, MUDRA AND CONCENTRATION.

125

THE YOGI WHO IS VIGILANT AND WHOSE MIND IS ONE POINTED IN SAMADHI WILL FIND RUDRANI OR SHAMBHAVI MUDRA MOST EFFECTIVE IN BESTOWING SIDDHIS.

126

ASANAS, PRANAYAMA, MUDRAS AND THIS WORLD WILL BE MEANINGLESS UNLESS ONE REACHES PERFECTION.

In other words, every stage of your practice should serve to take you to a higher stage until perfection is reached. No stage in your practice should be an end in itself. So when people get stuck in Asana practice, they are wasting their life if it does not serve a higher purpose.

127
THE YOGI SHOULD PRACTICE PRANAYAMA WITH A CONCENTRATED MIND AND SHOULD NOT LET IT WANDER.

128
THUS, THE TEN MUDRAS WERE TAUGHT BY ADINATH, SHAMBHU, AND EACH ONE IS CAPABLE OF BESTOWING PERFECTION TO THE YOGI.

This is very important to bear in mind. You do not have to be involved in all of the Mudra practices. Choose one that appeals to you and pursue it to the goal of perfection. To enter a house, you only need to go through one door.

129
HE ALONE IS A TRUE GURU AND IS REGARDED AS ISHVARA HIMSELF WHO IMPARTS THE TRADITIONAL TEACHING OF MUDRAS TO HIS DIS-CIPLES.

130
THE YOGI WHO FAITHFULLY PRACTICES MUDRA ACCORDING TO HIS GURU'S INSTRUCTIONS WILL OBTAIN ALL THE SIDDHIS LIKE ANIMA ETC. AND OVERCOME DEATH.

Chapter Four

SAMADHI

1

SALUTATIONS TO THE GURU SHIVA, WHO IS OF THE NATURE OF NADA, BINDU AND KALAA. THE YOGI WHO IS WHOLLY DEVOTED TO HIM REACHES THE HIGHEST STATE OF BLISS.

Shiva is "of the nature of" Nada, Bindu and Kalaa, just like Brahman is of the nature of Satchitananda. Nada is the cause of creation. Bindu is the point of origin and Kalaa is that which radiates. Although many commentators provide long explanations of these, it is difficult to express them in ordinary concepts that the mind can grasp. One needs to experience it in order to fully comprehend it.

2

NOW, I WILL EXPOUND ON THE BEST METHOD OF REACHING THAT HIGHEST STATE OF SAMADHI WHICH LEADS TO EVERLASTING PEACE AND BLISS.

3 – 4

RAJA YOGA, SAMADHI, UNMANI, MANONMANI, AMARATWA, LAYA, SAHA-JA, TATTVA, SHUNYASHUNYA, PARAMPADAM, AMANASKAM, ADWAITAM, NIRALAMBA, NIRANJANA, JIVANMUKTI AND TURIYA ARE ALL SYNONY-MOUS TERMS.

When you read these two Slokas, it is clearly evident that the use of the term Raja Yoga means the highest experience of Oness with the Supreme. They literally state that Raja Yoga is synonymous with Samadhi, Unmani, Manonmani, etc. And yet commentators have been steadfast in explaining that Hatha Yoga is merely a beginning preparation for the system of Raja Yoga. The term Raja Yoga is not used here to describe a system but rather a state of consciousness. It is simply astonishing how there can be any confusion about this when the Slokas are clear.

5

JUST AS SALT WHEN DISSOLVED IN WATER BECOMES ONE WITH IT, SO IS MIND WHEN MERGED IN THE SELF. THIS IS KNOWN AS SAMADHI.

If you want to know what Samadhi is, you must experience it. This description is only giving you an indication of Samadhi. The Slokas continue to provide other examples of the state of merging.

6
WHEN PRANA IS WITHOUT AGITATION, THE MIND BECOMES STILL AND THIS IS SAMADHI.

These Slokas are trying to explain Samadhi in various ways. All the pictures, imagery and ideas only give you an idea or indication of what Samadhi is, but in actuality, it is none of that. The system of Raja Yoga, in essence, conveys the same idea. When the mind is still, without agitation, you reach Samadhi because it is only then that you are identifying with who you are. It does not matter which system you are studying and practicing. Anyone of them should bring the mind to a state of steadiness because that is the goal. The less fluctuation in your mind, the more you experience who you are until you reach the state where there is no more thought, no more agitation and you abide in your true nature. Anything less or other than that complete steadiness of mind, means that you are identifying with thoughts, ideas, notions and fluctuations, not with your true Self.

7
WHEN THE YOGI EXPERIENCES THE IDENTITY OF THE INDIVIDUAL SOUL WITH THE SUPREME SOUL, ALL THOUGHTS DISAPPEAR. THIS IS KNOWN AS SAMADHI.

It is like saying, "Which comes first, the chicken or the egg?" Do all thoughts disappear when you experience your Oneness with the Supreme Soul? Or must you eradicate all thoughts first in order to experience your Oneness with the Supreme Soul? In reality, it does not matter how you see it or how you express it. The point is that Samadhi is a thoughtless state, without any modifications of the mind or any ideas.

8

ONLY THROUGH THE GRACE AND GUIDANCE OF THE GURU CAN THE YOGI ATTAIN RAJA YOGA, ENLIGHTENMENT, LIBERATION OR PERFEC-
TION.

9

RENUNCIATION, SELF-KNOWLEDGE AND SAMADHI ARE IMPOSSIBLE WITHOUT THE COMPASSION OF THE GURU.

Renunciation, self-knowledge and Samadhi are very subtle experiences, each of which occur at different stages and levels of one's evolution. What is renunciation? It is the practice of giving up and letting go of possessiveness. We relate to things as possessions, whether they be material objects or relationships: "my car, my job, my wife, my husband, my friend...." So it involves how you relate to everyone and everything that presents itself to you in this world.

While you are preoccupied with your friends, companions and associates in the world, there is no thought of renunciation. These are all acquisitions that you hold onto. You develop attachment to them until you go over the edge, sacrificing that which is most important for that which creates bondage. You lose all discrimination, which leads to further ignorance and bondage. The more you are attached to something or someone, the more agitation is created in your mind, which in turn, leads you further and further from the goal of liberation.

On a practical level, you cannot give up everything because the mind cannot live in a vacuum. Therefore you must substitute. Sacrifice and give up that which enslaves you for that which will free you. The whole world is based on the law of sacrifice, renouncing one thing for another. If you want to be free, then you have to let go of bondage. The world is constantly teaching you but you are blinded by ignorance and cannot see these lessons. Instead, you fight against it life after life, developing disease of the mind based on the notion that the more you are attached to the world, the more happiness you will experience. You continue headlong in this process until someone of knowledge, wisdom and right discrimination wakes you up to the fact that you are heading in the wrong direction.

So how do you turn around? For example, if you are driving a car, traveling north 90 miles per hour when you need to go south, how do you reverse direction? First, you must be convinced that you are heading in the wrong direction. Someone either has to tell you or you see a sign. Next, you must slow down. Then you can stop and turn around. You do not just suddenly turn the car around. But even when you are convinced that you are going the wrong way, sometimes you will continue because part of you still thinks you are headed in the right direction. This is where the Guru comes in.

A Guru possesses compassion, awareness and grace. He will convince you that you are headed in the wrong direction, which is the hardest thing for a spiritual aspirant to accept and assimilate. Once the aspirant accepts this, he begins to slow down, stop and turn around. Sometimes people refuse to receive that help, proclaiming, "I've gone too far. I can't turn back. I've reached the point of no return." But it is never too late to turn around.

This renunciation comes through the compassion of the Guru who will dare to tell you that you are on the wrong track and that you need to change what you are doing. He meets you where you are. Do not expect to wake up one day and give up the entire world. Reununciation happens in stages.

The state of renunciation arises when there is knowledge, understanding and dis-passion. You have to constantly develop dispassion. Dispassion arises when you see the imperfection in something. You discover that it is not really what it seems. It is unreal, like a mirage. You find that you are being duped. When you realize that you are being fooled, that you do not have the right understanding, that this is not the Reality or the Truth, you will want to abandon it. You may find that your mind is fooling you, society is fooling you, advertising is fooling you, etc. Being fooled means that the Reality is one thing and what you imagine and expect it to be is another thing. You expect to be happy and fulfilled but you do not find fulfillment in the things you chase.

If you buy a product and it fails to meet your expectation, what do you do? You return it. When you realize that your mind is fooling you, what do you do? Do you plead with God to give you another mind because you do not want this one? Where are you going to find God? Why is it that you cannot find God anywhere to exchange it? You seek and seek but you do not find God. It is because thou art that. Thou art God. Who will exchange it for you? You, yourself. Because you are that. Everything is expressing this basic truth to you. You created it. You are the one who gave it to yourself. You are the one who has to undo it. You cannot go to someone and say, "Please change my mind."

Renunciation, self knowledge and Samadhi are impossible without the compassion of a Guru. Self knowledge and Samadhi are not possible unless there is renunciation, meaning that you have to give up wrong notion, wrong thinking, wrong identification and unreality. You cannot have both. You cannot say, "I am wise" and still be fooled all the time.

10

BY THE DISCIPLINES OF VARIOUS ASANAS, KUMBHAKAS AND MUDRAS, KUNDALINI SHAKTI IS AWAKENED AND THE PRANA ENTERS SUSHUM-NA.

11

THE YOGI WHOSE SHAKTI IS AWAKENED AND WHO IS ESTABLISHED IN RENUNCIATION ATTAINS SAMADHI.

Here, you can discern that there is a process you must undergo to attain Samadhi. You prepare for it by being involved in all these disciplines, such as Asanas, Kumbhakas, Mudras and renunciation. You must discipline your senses and mind. To do this, you must start with the basics. Since you can relate easily to the body, work with that first. Do not start from the point of Samadhi because it would be impossible for you to understand it. Similarly, if you want to write a book, you cannot start by publishing it. You have to write it first. It is a step-by-step process. Everybody wants to write a book but they do not have any idea how to do it. In fact, often they do not even have any ideas. If you ask them, "What are you writing a book about?" The response is, "I don't know but I'll write a book." How many children do not know their ABC's but when they open a book, they are convinced that they are reading?

It is the same thing with Samadhi. First, you must begin with basic disciplines. The Yogi performs various Asanas, Kumbhakas and Mudras. Then the Shakti is awakened and Prana enters the Sushumna. The Yogi whose Shakti is awakened and who is established in renunciation attains Samadhi. You must go through the process where there is less and less identification with unreality and you are moving closer to a state of freedom through renunciation.

12

WHEN PRANA FLOWS THROUGH SUSHUMNA AND THE MIND IS IN THE STATE OF SHUNYA, THE YOGI IS FREED FROM THE EFFECTS OF KARMA.

Karma means action. Every action calls forth an effect or reaction. The whole universe is based on this law of cause and effect. As Jesus said, "As you sow, so shall you reap." How then could the Yogi be freed from the effects of Karma? The individual experiences this world of time, space and causation in the three states of waking, dreaming and deep sleep. In these states, one is subject to the law of Karma because one is identifying with mind, body, intellect and the world of change. But from the Absolute standpoint, one is not this mind, body and intellect, and this world of change is not the reality. So Karma is really wrong identification. When you arrogate action to yourself, then you have to reap the fruits of your action. The Self, the Soul, the Atman does not act. It is really the three Gunas that are acting. The Self is simply the experiencer and the mind, body and intellect are the instruments that are involved in action. In the state of Shunya, the Yogi experiences his identity with the Higher Reality and realizes that he is the Self, the Soul, the Atman. Thus, he is freed from the effects of Karma. This is a state of enlightenment.

13

SALUTATIONS OH IMMORTAL ONE FOR YOU HAVE MASTERED TIME. YOU INTO WHOSE JAWS THE ANIMATE AND INANIMATE HAVE BEEN DEVOURED.

The Yogi becomes immortal and is worthy of salutation and reverence because he has mastered time. He has gone beyond the relative state of understanding and identification, beyond duality, space and time.

14

WHEN AMAROLI, VAJROLI AND SAHAJOLI ARE MASTERED, PRANA
ENTERS THE SUSHUMNA AND THE MIND BECOMES CALM.

15

SELF KNOWLEDGE AND LIBERATION ARE NOT POSSIBLE AS LONG AS
MIND AND PRANA ARE FLUCTUATING.

These Slokas, in essence, are just repeating the same thing. Liberation and self
knowledge are other ways to state the goal of Yoga. That goal can never be reached
as long as the Prana or the mind is fluctuating. Mind and Prana are interrelated
so that when one fluctuates, the other fluctuates. Self knowledge and liberation
are an effect or a state that is reached when the mind and Prana become steady.

16

BEING IN THE RIGHT ENVIRONMENT AND HAVING LEARNED HOW TO
PIERCE THE SUSHUMNA, MAKE THE PRANA FLOW AND REMAIN IN THIS
CENTER OF HIGHER CONSCIOUSNESS.

17

DAY AND NIGHT ARE ASSOCIATED WITH THE SUN AND THE MOON.
THE GREAT SECRET IS THAT THE SUSHUMNA CONSUMES TIME.

When consciousness flows through Sushumna, then duality ceases for the Yogi.

18

THERE ARE 72,000 NADIS IN THE BODY. OF THESE, SUSHUMNA IS THE
MOST IMPORTANT.

All these Nadis or tributaries lead to one river called Sushumna, which is the most
important one.

19
WHEN KUNDALINI IS AWAKENED, BOTH PRANA AND KUNDALINI CAN ENTER SUSHUMNA WITHOUT OBSTRUCTION.

20
THE STATE OF MANONMANI IS REACHED WHEN PRANA FLOWS THROUGH SUSHUMNA OTHERWISE ALL OTHER PRACTICES WILL BE USELESS.

Manonmani means the state of no mind. It is reached when the Prana flows through Sushumna. The phrase, "otherwise all other practices will be useless," means that unless your practice is leading you to the purification of Sushumna where Prana will flow unobstructed, then it is not a useful, constructive practice. Your practice should result in focus, concentration and purity of mind.

21
THROUGH THE CONTROL OF PRANA, THE MIND IS CONTROLLED AND THE YOGI THAT HAS CONTROL OF HIS MIND HAS CONTROL OF PRANA ALSO.

22
MIND IS AN EFFECT OF VASANAS AND PRANA, IF ONE IS CONTROLLED, THE OTHER IS CONTROLLED ALSO.

What is mind? It is the fluctuation of Prana and Vasanas, which are thoughts. Mind can be defined as a bundle of thoughts. When there is no thought, there is no mind. Mind is the effect of the movement of Vasanas and Prana. If you can control the mind, then you can control Prana and vice versa

23
WHEN THE BREATH IS CONTROLLED, THE MIND IS SUSPENDED AND WHEN MIND IS CONTROLLED, THE BREATH IS SUSPENDED.

This is self-explanatory. The Sutras are written in such a way that they do not have to be expounded on here.

24

THIS INTERRELATIONSHIP OF MIND AND PRANA IS LIKE A MIXTURE OF MILK AND WATER. THUS, WHEN MIND IS ACTIVE, PRANA IS ACTIVE AND VICE VERSA.

How can you separate one from the other? You cannot separate milk from water. They are both interrelated. They are one and the same.

25

THEREFORE, BY SUSPENDING ONE, THE OTHER BECOMES SUSPENDED AND BY ACTIVATING ONE, THE OTHER BECOMES ACTIVE AND ALL THE SENSES BECOME ALIVE. MOSKSHA OR LIBERATION IS REACHED WHEN THEY ARE BROUGHT UNDER CONTROL.

When the Prana is active, you will find that all the senses are alive. When this happens, there is externalization, fluctuation and agitation of the mind, so that you are not experiencing the ultimate truth. You are moving further away from the Reality. When you control the Prana and the mind, then withdrawal is taking place. With practice, Pratyahara takes place through withdrawing, thus enabling you to reach back to the source.

26

MERCURY AND MIND ARE BY NATURE UNSTEADY. WHAT ON EARTH IS THERE THAT CANNOT BE ATTAINED IF ONE CAN GAIN CONTROL OF THESE?

Mercury is a tangible thing that one can relate to. It is by nature unsteady, but it is possible to make it steady. If you understand how to bring the mind into steadiness, just as you can steady mercury, then there is nothing you cannot attain in this world.

27

OH PARVATI, WHEN MERCURY AND BREATH ARE MADE STEADY, ALL DISEASES ARE ERADICATED, THE DEAD BECOME ALIVE AND ONE MOVES IN SPACE.

Some people read this and fantasize that if they can control mercury then they will be able to fly in space. They become involved in witchcraft, voodoo, alchemy and all kinds of unwise practices without understanding that the Sloka is really referring to the mind. This misunderstanding leads to all kinds of superstition. For example, people believe that if they wear a certain talisman, ring or crystal, it will confer certain powers on them and allow them to perform supernatural feats. Thus the mind is made to move outward rather than inward. As a result, the mind becomes dependent on external forces. Since people will often exploit this weakness, why leave yourself susceptible?

28

WHEN MIND IS STEADY, THE BREATH AND BINDU BECOME STEADY. THE STEADINESS OF BINDU RESULTS IN A SATTWIC AND STEADY BODY.

The Bindu is expressed as the creative force or the seed. It has a tendency to move out to express itself to unite with its counterpart, such as the semen seeking to unite with the ovum so that something else will sprout from it. All these tendencies within you are designed to keep you in constant bondage. It maintains your mind in a state of agitation. If you look at the type of movies people watch today, it reflects a base consciousness, stirring up the sexual energy and violence. This is the accepted norm, reflecting the life of most people today. They have no higher aspiration because they do not know of any. There is no Guru to guide them. The closest thing to a Guru for most people is their parents, who are also confused and corrupted by wrong conditioning since it is propagated from generation to generation without right understanding or right knowledge. One of the greatest blessings in life is to have a Guru who can guide you.

When the breath and Bindu become steady. This results in a Sattwic and steady body. Thus, you want the Bindu to be steady. Why try to agitate it? Why stir it up?

29
MIND IS THE MASTER OF THE SENSES AND PRANA IS THE MASTER OF THE MIND. LAYA IS THE LORD OF PRANA AND LAYA DEPENDS ON NADA.

This outlines the order of importance of these forces. From this you know that you can control the senses by the mind and that the mind can be brought under control by gaining control of Prana. The state of Laya is reached when both mind and Prana is steady. In that stillness Nada is experienced which becomes the cause for greater or deeper stillness.

30
THIS IS CALLED MOKSHA BUT OTHERS MAY DISAGREE. HOWEVER, WHEN MIND AND PRANA ARE IN LAYA, AN INDESCRIBABLE BLISS IS EXPERIENCED.

31
THE YOGI IS IN A STATE OF LAYA OR ABSORPTION WHEN THE MIND AND SENSES ARE UNDER CONTROL.

32
WHEN ALL THOUGHTS AND ACTIONS CEASE, THIS RESULTS IN LAYA WHICH IS KNOWN ONLY BY ONESELF AND IS BEYOND WORDS.

With respect to these higher states of being, it is difficult to explain or convey the idea to someone. Even though you can intellectualize and philosophize about it, there is still no actual experience. For example, if you wanted to learn about the lightbulb and electricity, I could explain all the theories and laws that govern electricity but you will never experience it other than through the light. If I told you that electricity shocks you, what does that mean? You would have to practice electricity Yoga and push your finger in the socket to experience it. Just like electrical shock, Laya is "beyond words."

33
THE MIND MERGES IN THE OBJECT OF CONCENTRATION. THE ELEMENTS, SENSES AND PRANA EXIST ETERNALLY IN ALL LIVING BEINGS AND ARE ABSORBED IN BRAHMAN.

You must go through the process of Pratyahara (withdrawal of the senses), Dharana (concentration) and Dhyana (meditation) until it leads you into that state of transcendence.

34
WHAT IS MEANT BY THE EXPRESSION LAYA, LAYA? IT IS THE NON-APPREHENSION OF OBJECTS DUE TO THE CESSATION OF VASANAS.

Objects appear to be one thing or another according to the fluctuation or modification of the mind. Once the Vasanas cease and the Prana stops, there is absorption or apprehension of the Reality and non-apprehension of objects which is otherwise known as Laya.

SHAMBHAVI MUDRA

35
THE VEDAS, SHASTRAS AND PURANAS ARE LIKE COMMON WOMEN BUT SHAMBHAVI IS RESERVED LIKE A WOMAN OF REFINED CULTURE.

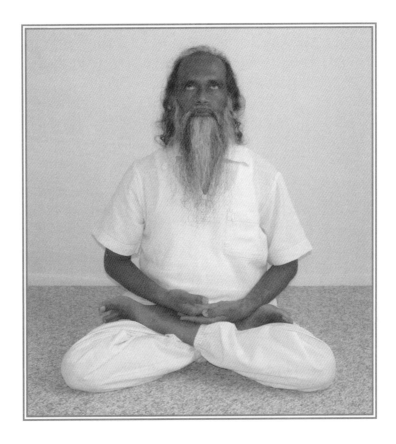

36
WITH THE MIND INTERNALIZED AND ONE-POINTED AND THE EXTERNAL GAZE UNBLINKING, THIS IS SHAMBHAVI MUDRA PRESERVED IN THE VEDAS AND SHASTRAS.

37
WHEN THE MIND AND PRANA ARE ABSORBED IN THE SELF AND THE GAZE IS MOTIONLESS, THIS IS SHAMBHAVI MUDRA. THE STATE OF SHUNYASHUNYA ARISES WHEN THIS IS GIVEN WITH THE GRACE OF THE GURU. THIS IS THE REAL STATE OF SHIVA.

38

EVEN THOUGH THE PLACE OF CONCENTRATION AND INFLUENCE OF SRI SHAMBHAVI AND KHECHARI ARE DIFFERENT, THEY BOTH RESULT IN CHIT SUKHA, BLISSFUL EXISTENCE.

In Khechari, you focus on the place where the point of the three rivers, Ida, Pingala and Sushumna, converge by taking the tongue back. In Shambhavi, you focus on the point between the eyebrows. The result is the same in both Mudras: purification of the mind, Chit Sukha, blissful existence.

U N M A N I

39

WITH THE ATTENTION ON THE LIGHT BETWEEN THE EYEBROWS BY RAISING THE EYEBROWS A LITTLE AS IN THE PREVIOUS PRACTICE, THE YOGI SOON REACHES THE STATE OF UNMANI.

If you practice Shambhavi Mudra, keeping the attention at the point between the eyebrows, a light will appear. If you continue to concentrate on that light, the state of Unmani arises.

40

SOME FOLLOW THE AGAMAS WHILE OTHERS ARE CAUGHT UP IN THE NIGAMAS AND LOGIC BUT NONE OF THEM KNOW THE WAY TO LIBERATION.

All the Scriptures, the Agamas and Nigamas, are based on logics and reasoning. People get caught up in the fine points of logics and reasoning but they really do not know what liberation is. It is beyond all of these things. Even though they lead one to the doorway, one has to step through, which takes faith and courage. Trust and unshakable faith in the Guru facilitates this.

41

THE YOGI SITTING MOTIONLESS AND GAZING AT THE TIP OF THE
NOSE WITH EYES HALF CLOSED AND BY STOPPING THE MOVEMENT OF
IDA AND PINGALA, EXPERIENCES THAT LIGHT WHICH IS ENDLESS,
COMPLETE, RADIANT AND SUPREME. WHAT MORE IS THERE TO BE
SAID?

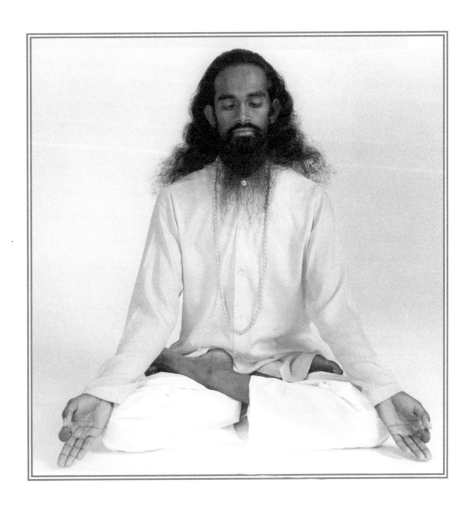

42

THE ATMAN IS WORSHIPPED NEITHER BY DAY NOR NIGHT. ONLY BY SUSPENDING IDA AND PINGALA IS THE ATMAN WORSHIPPED.

The state of experiencing the Atman, the Self, is not a relative state. While Prana flows through the Ida and Pingala, night and day, you are experiencing the state of duality and it is not really the Atman that is being worshipped. Rather, it is your own fantasy and notion of what reality is. You believe that God is one thing or another and you project that onto your experience. The phrase, "The Atman is worshipped by neither day nor night," means that it is beyond our imagination and comprehension. It is beyond description and explanation. It is only by suspending Ida and Pingala or going beyond duality, that the Atman is worshipped, which means that you are in constant awareness of the Self.

KHECHARI MUDRA

43

KHECHARI MUDRA IS SUCCESSFUL WHEN THE PRANA LEAVES IDA AND PINGALA AND FLOWS THROUGH SUSHUMNA.

44

THE YOGI BECOMES ESTABLISHED IN KHECHARI MUDRA WHEN THE PRANA, ENTERING SUSHUMNA, BECOMES MOTIONLESS.

45

THAT MUDRA KNOWN AS KHECHARI IS PERFORMED IN THE UNSUP-PORTED SPACE WHICH IS BETWEEN THE IDA AND PINGALA AND IS CALLED VYOMA CHAKRA.

46

THE OPENING OF THE DIVINE SUSHUMNA IS FILLED FROM BEHIND WITH THE NECTAR THAT FLOWS FROM CHANDRA, SHIVA'S BELOVED.

47

THE SUSHUMNA BEING COMPLETELY FILLED LEADS TO UNMANI.

48

THE POINT BETWEEN THE EYEBROWS IS THE SEAT OF SHIVA. WHEN THE MIND BECOMES ABSORBED THERE, THE TIMELESS STATE, TURIYA, IS EXPERIENCED.

The same truth is repeated here. The state of Khechari is not achieved simply by cutting the tongue and pulling it out. These are practices designed to take you to the point where the Prana enters the Sushumna and the mind becomes motionless. It is similar to saying that Pranayama is not merely breathing exercises. But through such practices, you will reach the point where you can control the Prana.

49

TIME IS NON-EXISTENT FOR THE YOGI WHO PRACTICES THE KHECHARI UNTIL YOGA NIDRA IS ATTAINED.

Yoga Nidra is Yogic sleep, which means that you are no longer identifying with modifications. When you enter that state of Yoga Nidra, time is nonexistent, just like in deep sleep. There is no time in Yoga Nidra and Samadhi.

50

THE YOGI, SITTING WITHOUT A THOUGHT, IS LIKE AN EMPTY POT FILLED INSIDE AND OUTSIDE WITH SPACE.

What is Samadhi? It is a state without thought, filled in silence. Here the Sloka draws another analogy. No matter where you move an empty pot, it is always pervaded by space. Similarly, only when there is no thought will the Yogi experience the Supreme Consciousness. Then he abides in his real nature of Sat-Chit-Ananda. While there is thought, he identifies with the thought waves.

51
**WHEN PRANA AND THE MIND ARE SUSPENDED, THE EXTERNAL
BREATH IS ALSO SUSPENDED.**

This is Nada Kumbhaka. My Guru, Swami Nada-Brahmananda was able to do
this for 37 minutes. People mistakenly thought he was holding his breath. But, in
actuality, the breath was suspended. Nada Kumbhaka is an effect of suspending
the Prana and the mind. It is not something that you do but rather a state that
you reach. If you try to hold your breath for 37 minutes, you will fail.

52
**BY REGULAR PRACTICE, PRANA AND MIND ARE BROUGHT UNDER CON-
TROL.**

Prana and mind are brought under control by regular practice, not simply by
Shaktipat when the Guru touches you on the forehead or through a secret formula or Mantra.

53
**THE YOGI POSSESSES A SUPERIOR BODY WITH SUPERIOR STRENGTH
AND IMMENSE VALOR WHEN THE WHOLE BODY IS FILLED WITH NEC-
TAR FROM THE HEAD TO THE FEET.**

54
**MERGING THE MIND IN KUNDALINI AND KUNDALINI IN THE MIND,
OBSERVE THE MIND WITH THE MIND AND CONTEMPLATE THE HIGHER
REALITY.**

55
**MERGING ATMAN IN BRAHMAN AND BRAHMAN IN ATMAN, EXPERIENC-
ING BRAHMAN EVERYWHERE, REMAIN IN THAT STATE WITHOUT
THOUGHT.**

56

THE YOGI EXPERIENCES BRAHMAN INSIDE AND OUTSIDE JUST LIKE AN EMPTY POT IN THE OCEAN.

Just like the empty pot in space, the same analogy is given with the empty pot in the ocean. When the individual is empty of the ego and false identification of body, mind, etc., he experiences the pervasiveness of Brahman as the empty pot in the ocean.

57

THE YOGI ABANDONING ALL THOUGHT, REMAINS IN THAT STATE.

58

OH RAMA, THE ENTIRE UNIVERSE IS NOTHING BUT A PROJECTION OF THE MIND AND MIND IS NOTHING BUT THOUGHTS. WHEN THOUGHTS SUBSIDE, THE YOGI EXPERIENCES PEACE.

This Sloka indicates that Swatamarama draws from the teachings of the different Masters like Sage Vashishta's discourse to Lord Rama, known as *The Yoga Vashishta*, to explain the experience of Samadhi or enlightenment.

59

THE MIND DISSOLVES IN SAMADHI JUST AS CAMPHOR DISAPPEARS IN FIRE AND SALT DISSOLVES IN WATER.

60

DUALITY DISAPPEARS WHEN THE KNOWER, KNOWLEDGE AND THE KNOWN BECOME ONE.

61

THE WHOLE WORLD OF ANIMATE OR INANIMATE IS NOTHING BUT THE MODIFICATION OF THE MIND. IN THE STATE OF UNMANI, THERE IS NO DUALITY.

62

THE STATE OF KAIVALYA IS REACHED WHEN THERE IS NO MODIFICATION OF THE MIND.

63

THUS, THE ANCIENT MASTERS HAVING DIRECT EXPERIENCE OF THE HIGHER REALITY EXPLAINED THE VARIOUS METHODS OF REACHING THERE.

There are various methods to experience the higher reality as explained by the ancient Masters. These include Kumbhakas, Mudras, etc. They come from different Masters who used such methods to realize the Self. This is the reason why one person practicing Tantric Yoga may be performing Vajroli Mudra and another person may be practicing Khechari. It does not matter which path you take as long as it leads you safely to the ultimate goal.

64

SALUTATIONS TO THEE OH SUSHUMNA, KUNDALINI, MANONMANI, THE NECTAR FLOWING FROM THE MOON, THE GREAT SHAKTI AND THE ATMAN.

The different ways of expressing the state of Samadhi by different names probably stems from different Masters. In Sloka 58, you find the phrase "Oh Rama," which is from *The Yoga Vasistha*, in which Rama and his Guru, Vasistha, discuss the nature of reality using the pot analogy. All these analogies are a projection of the mind. From these different minds derive all different expressions of Samadhi. But the actual experience of the Higher Reality in that transcendental state remains the same.

NADA YOGA

65

I WILL NOW DESCRIBE THE PRACTICE OF NADA YOGA AS EXPOUNDED BY GORAKSHANATH WHICH IS UNDERSTANDABLE TO EVEN THE UNEDUCATED WHO IS INCAPABLE OF COMPREHENDING THE PHILOSOPHY OF THE HIGHER REALITY.

Nada Yoga has its roots in the Vedas. It is the science of Divine vibration, as revealed to the Mystics, Saints and Yogis who have used it to reach Self-Realization, the experience of Oneness with Brahman, the Supreme Consciousness. Nada Yoga involves a tuning into subtler vibrations, one's internal music and sounds, until ultimately, one reaches a state where there is absolute silence and peace, returning to the source of creation, to God. This state is attainable by an individual who has reached a high level of purification through his Sadhana.

Although many have attempted to dissect and analyze Nada Yoga, it is not just an intellectual pursuit but rather an experiential one. That is why the Nada Yogi delves into the practice without having to fully understand it, striving for the state that will lead to complete absorption and experience.

The vehicle for its transmission is Indian classical music in the form of Ragas, Talas, Slokas, Mantras, chanting, Kirtan and Bhajans. One does not have to be an established Nada Yogi or learned in Vedanta philosophy to practice. Anyone can be involved in this, whether educated or uneducated, so long as they chant the name of God with love and devotion. This practice will help to purify the body, mind, emotions and intellect, creating transformation so that one can tune into the subtler internal vibrations.

66

EVEN THOUGH ADINATH TAUGHT MORE THAN ONE AND A QUARTER CRORES OF METHODS TO REACH LAYA, I CONSIDER THE EXPLORATION OF ANAHATA NADA TO BE THE BEST.

The phrase, "one and a quarter crores," literally means one and a quarter of ten million. Its use here illustrates that there are innumerable ways given by Adinath, also known as Shiva or God, to reach Laya or Samadhi. Whatever method employed, the individual must undergo an intense purification of the body, mind, senses, intellect and ego. Of all the different methods taught, Yogi Swatmarama considers Anahata Nada to be the best.

The question naturally arises, "Why is it the best?" The aim of all Yoga paths is to refine the whole personality so that the light of the Divine Self shines through in all its splendor. Ultimately every form of Yoga, whether it is Hatha Yoga, Raja Yoga, Karma Yoga, Bhakti Yoga, Jnana Yoga, etc., if practiced earnestly and with unwavering discipline, will culminate in Nada Yoga, the experience of the Anahata Nada. The different paths of Yoga are designed to suit different personalities. While the best Yoga practice is one that integrates the various paths, such as Sampoorna Yoga, someone with a natural sense of music will obviously have a proclivity to place more emphasis on the aspect of Nada Yoga. But it is not just for the musically inclined. Nada Yoga uses Divine music to move from the gross differentiated vibrations to the subtlest state until it reaches the source. It enchants and stills the mind so that it becomes completely absorbed in Divine vibration, which is the essence underlying all of creation.

Moreover, the practice of Asana, Pranayama, Kriyas, proper diet and positive thinking can be used as components of Nada Yoga because they all deal with energy and vibration. Each practice helps to tune and refine the instrument of perception until the goal of Yoga is reached. A sick person is unable to sing because his instrument, the body, is not properly tuned. To sing, one must be free from congestion and be able to breathe properly, which naturally involves modifying one's diet and avoiding foods that generate an excess of mucus in the system. The practice of Asana, Pranayama, Kriyas and observance of pure diet tunes up all the systems, enhances the purification and refinement process, which will ultimately lead to the experience of Anahata Nada.

So what does Swatmarama mean by the "exploration of the Anahata Sound?" First, it helps to understand what Divine vibration is. The Bible declares, "In the beginning was the Word and the Word was with God and the Word was God and the word became manifest." The statement implies that the universe is nothing but an expression and manifestation of the Divine. God is not in the universe but the universe is God. Whether something is manifest in the physical, astral or causal world, animate or inanimate, seen or unseen, perceived or unperceived, it all constitutes Brahman as vibration.

According to the Vedas, Brahman, the One without a second, manifests as this universe in the form of vibration, which modern scientists refer to as the big bang. The first manifestation of the Absolute is referred to as "Om," Pranava or Nada Brahman. This is the Para state, which is the most subtle undifferentiated vibration, the immutable essence underlying all of creation. While this concept is elusive and difficult to grasp with our limited intellect, Vedanta and Samkhya philosophy provide some insight.

When the creative aspect of Brahman becomes many, its energy aspect, Prakriti (the term used in Vedanta and Samkhya philosophy) or Shakti (the term used in

Tantric tradition) manifests as this universe. Prakriti or Shakti is nature, the Divine Mother, and descends into this creation from the most subtle to the gross. From the Para state, this primordial energy interacting with Purusha, which is pure consciousness, becomes more differentiated and manifests into the three Gunas, which are the three inseparable forces expressed in all of creation. They are: Sattwa, a state of balance; Rajas, a state of activity and movement; and Tamas a state of inertia or darkness. This level of manifestation is still subtle and is referred to as the Pashyanti state. The three Gunas, in their subtle state, are in the transcendental realm, which is beyond the ability of mind and intellect to grasp. Therefore, one can only experience it in the transcendental state through meditation. As these Gunas begin to combine with one another, the state of mental vibration, known as the Madhyama state, is created. Here, one can relate to the vibration in the form of universal concepts. For example, when you think of water, regardless of what your language, culture, or geographpical location, the mental concept of water, the liquid that quenches your thirst, will still be the same. No matter how you express it in words or sounds, the concept is still the same. The last state is the Vaikhari state, in which this world of objects, names and forms, sound, language and music can be perceived through the senses, which of course, are interpreted by the mind.

Thus, everything in the universe comes from vibration, and in its essence, is vibration (or energy). Vibration as sound exists in many different forms, ranging from the very gross to the extremely subtle. Even our physical body (made up of the elements), astral body (comprised of the energy, mental and intellectual sheaths) and our causal body (comprised of the blissful sheath) are vibration. For example, the energy system, known as the Pranamaya Kosha, is made up of the Nadis and

Chakra system, which are receptors of vibration and mostly influenced by sound vibration. This is why music has such a strong effect on us. If you understand this, you will understand why it is so important to expose yourself to Divine vibration. The person of right discrimination will want to be influenced in a positive way rather than in a negative way.

Since every aspect of our being is greatly influenced by sound vibration, the ancient Masters formulated the system of Nada Yoga, starting with the audible level (Vaikhari state) to which we can most easily relate, for purification and Self-Realization. Nada Yoga is a very practical science because it addresses our very essence.

Nada Yoga refines and attunes all the bodily systems, the Nadis (the subtle channels through which energy flows), the mind and the intellect through sound vibration using external instruments such as the Veena, the Sarangi, the Sitar, the Guitar, the Sarod, the Harmonium or the Tabla. The body and the voice are the greatest instruments. One may study and learn the technical notes, Talas and Ragas, but it is for the sole purpose of transformation and Self-Realization. While singing or playing an instrument, one develops focus, concentration and absorption. Once the bodily equipment (physical, pranic, mental, intelletual and egoic systems) is refined and purified and the mind gradually becomes internalized, one is taken to higher levels of awareness and consciousness until ultimately, the individual consciousness realizes its Oneness with the Supreme Consciousness and the goal of Yoga is reached. As the mind becomes still and internalized, one experiences the Nadam, vibration, including the subtle movement of Prana and the Anahata sound, one's internal music, which is a means to take you to the state of

Samadhi. At that stage, the external instrument becomes redundant. This refinement and purification of the personality is a step-by-step process and takes many years of dedicated practice to reach that advanced state.

Through the practice of Nada Yoga, one undergoes a multidimensional transformation of all the systems and the ego. But for this to take place, devotion and humility must be firmly established or one will not be able to learn anything higher or sublime. An aspirant who sits in front of a Guru with an inflated ego will not learn anything because he is already full of himself and one must first empty his cup in order for it to be filled. Such a person will merely gather some information and techniques that would be used to further magnify his ego. No transformation would take place in his personality.

I studied for 14 years with my Guru, Swami Nada-Brahmananda, who was a Master of Nada Yoga. Most of his teachings were practical and experiential, starting from the most basic level. I did not spend innumerable hours pouring over books before delving into the practice. The truth is that the quantity of books one reads does not determine one's evolution. In fact, if not done with proper guidance, it might create wrong conditioning and hamper one's evolution. Some people gather all sorts of information but it is only what is put into practice that is of use. The rest of the information is only a distraction for the mind. Information by itself does not bring about transformation. That is why Master Sivananda said, "An ounce of practice is worth more than tons of theory."

Thus, one should pursue the path of transformation, continuing the disciplines of purification and refinement through Nada Yoga, so that one may eventually experience the Anahata sound. What is the Anahata sound? It is something distinct and different from the Ahata Nada. Ahata Nada is sound vibration that is experienced on the sensual level. For example, if someone strikes a drum, that vibration will travel through the air into the hearing mechanism in your body and you will hear the drum beat. The Anahata Nada, however, is experienced in the state of meditation as the subtle vibrations of Prana. With the mind internalized, one can hear an unstruck sound. In other words, the experience of the Anahata Nada does not require an external instrument to hear it.

There are different levels of unfoldment in the experience of Anahata Nada. Successively, one will hear chinne chinne, the sound of the ocean, the kunch, the kettledrums, the drum, the lute, the flute, the harp and the clapping of thunder. In the practice of Hatha Yoga, as the Granthis are pierced, different sounds or vibrations are experienced, as explained in subsequent Slokas. But do not stop there because they are not the ultimate goal. They are just stages that are reached in one's spiritual development. Every successive level is a sign that one is delving deeper and deeper within. The sounds charm the mind to dive into deeper levels of consciousness until one is able to pierce through the last veil and experience the Self without any conditioning.

"Gunghata ke pata khool re toe hai piyaa mileenge."

In other words, "Remove the veil and behold the Lord everywhere." God or Brahman is omnipresent, all pervading. The veils are our conditionings that we acquire by virtue of birth, culture, religion, environment, time, sex, age, education, level of intelligence and experience. All these identifications are veils, just like the body, mind, senses, intellect and emotions. The Higher Reality lies beyond all these conditionings. When the last veil is shattered, the Self is revealed in its full splendor. This state is called Samadhi, Turiya, the fourth state of consciousness, Self-Realization or God-Realization, Raja Yoga, Unmani, etc.

The reason why Indian classical music is the vehicle for the practice of Nada Yoga is because it has been perfected already. It was not developed but instead flowed through the minds of purified beings. It is the knowledge of the universe, knowledge of the Vedas. Veda literally means pure and perfect knowledge. The knowledge about Nada Yoga, which is contained in the Sama Veda, has been handed down from Guru to disciple as a systematic science. Since this knowledge is already perfect, nothing can be added to it.

In the West, people often think that Yoga has to be developed. Many think that just because they go into a certain posture or stretch that they are expanding the knowledge of Yoga. But this is delusion. People tend to get stuck on the superficial aspect of Yoga without the right perspective of the goal of Yoga. Therefore, there should be right knowledge, proper understanding and proper guidance from a Guru who will ensure that one is truly practicing Yoga, whether it is Hatha Yoga, Nada Yoga or any other spiritual discipline, for the purpose of reaching liberation. Nada Yoga is a systematic, step-by-step science, just like Hatha Yoga or any other Yoga for that matter.

> *Gaana Vidya Badikatinahe Janeto. Guru Charana Shisya Dhare.*
> *Tapa Vaave Mahaa Deva. Aadhi Devo Maha Deva. Veena Bajaa*
> *Tava. Tatabitata baaje.*

Translated, this Bhajan means: "Knowledge of music is very difficult to learn. You have to sit at the feet of the Guru, do Tapas and practice intense Sadhana. The first god is Maha Deva. He is the one who plays the Veena." According to legend, Lord Shiva strung the Veena with his veins. In other words, this universe is nothing but the body of the Lord and this music is present everywhere as vibration. It is no wonder why Swatmarama considers the exploration of Anahata Nada to be the best.

The knowledge of Nada Yoga was handed down from Guru to disciple. The source of it is God, divinity. The music people produce is an expression of their consciousness at that time. If the mind is polluted and corrupted, the music will reflect such pollution and corruption. If the mind is on a lower emotional state or immersed in sensuality, the music expressed through it will be accordingly. It would not be Nada Yoga because it would not lead one to a higher level of consciousness. In fact, such music will only serve to create more agitation in the mind. It is very important to know the basic distinction between music that is uplifting and music that keeps one on a lower state of consciousness.

When vibration is flowing through the harmonized mind of a Yogi, Divine music is produced. Such music is healing and lifts the consciousness out of a state of restlessness, anxiety and depression to a state of calmness, peacefulness and bliss. With this fundamental understanding, one practices music with a different state of awareness. That is when music becomes sacred. It becomes Yoga and helps people to evolve, grow and refine.

Many musicians may practice Indian classical music and are considered accomplished but that does not necessarily mean that they are practicing Nada Yoga. If they perform merely for entertainment, they are boosting their ego, thereby creating an even thicker veil. Only when music is practiced to transform the personality with a view to becoming more refined and humble, can it be called Nada Yoga. So the kind of music one produces should bring one to a state of Sattwa or balance so that one can experience one's Divinity. In order to do this, there must be purification of body, mind, intellect and ego. A Sattwic mind will produce Sattwic music, which will uplift the mind and create happiness, peace and bliss. Chanting and Kirtan performed by Yogis is an exmple of this. A Rajasic mind will express Rajisic music, which will only excite the mind and senses. An example of this is disco and nightclub music. A Tamasic mind will express Tamasic music, which will dull, degrade and corrupt the mind, senses and personality. For example, lamenting music that sends somone into depression is Tamasic. Everything one does should be for the purpose of positive transformation and refinement of the personality.

Every form of Yoga is for higher transformation. Nada Yoga reaches a point where it becomes so abstract that only the practitioner or the Yogi delights in or understands it. At that stage, it becomes internalized and personalized because it is for his own transformation. The more the Yogi becomes established and refined, the less people will be able to relate to his music because it becomes very abstract.

For example, my Guru, Swami Nada-Brahmananda, a great Master of Nada Yoga, gave a presentation but only a few people attended and some even left midway through because they did not understand what was taking place. They were unable to relate to it because they were vibrating at a lower level of consciousness. Unfortunately, this is the state of the world and existing consciousness today. Spiritual evolution is not measured by popularity. A musician is only popular if he caters to the consciousness of the masses. Having myself experienced the grandeur of the Divine gifts of Nada Yoga, I can only encourage you to explore this enlightened path. Simply put, it is music for the soul.

SHAMBHAVI MUDRA

67
SITTING IN MUKTASANA AND PERFORMING SHAMBHAVI MUDRA, THE YOGI SHOULD LISTEN ATTENTIVELY TO THE NADA WITHIN THE RIGHT EAR.

Here, the Yogi is instructed to perform Shambhavi Mudra and listen. Everybody can do this, whether they are an intellectual giant or a peasant in the field. Once there is purification, the individual, irrespective of his station in life, will be able to listen to the subtle sounds of Nada. In fact, the unlettered person is likely to have less agitation and delusion than the so-called educated individual. Most people in the West watch television every day, listening to nonsense, commercials, debates and movie reviews. It is a reflection of the shallowness of society. There is nothing else to talk about or to occupy the mind, even though we praise ourselves to be intellectuals. The result is a scattering of the mind with useless information.

68

THUS WITH THE EARS, NOSE AND MOUTH CLOSED, A CLEAR AND DISTINCT SOUND IS HEARD IN THE PURIFIED SUSHUMNA.

Not just anybody who closes their ears, nose, eyes and mouth will hear something. In actuality, the average person who does this will hear nothing. But the individual with a purified Sushumna will hear a clear distinct sound.

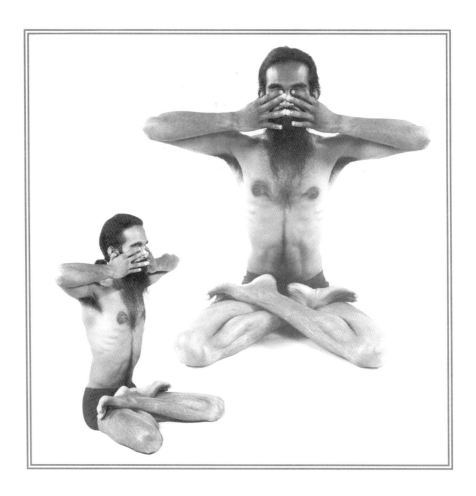

69

ALL YOGIC PRACTICES GO THROUGH FOUR STAGES: ARAMBHA, GHATA, PARICHAYA AND NISHPATTI.

In all practices, Arambha, Ghata, Parichaya and Nishpatti are the four stages encountered as you evolve to higher levels of consciousness. If you want to delve into the higher realms and the higher practices, you will go through these four stages.

ARAMBHA AVASTHA

70

WHEN THE BRAHMA GRANTHI IS PIERCED, THE YOGI EXPERIENCES BLISS AND THE ANAHATA SOUND OF TINKLING.

71

IN THIS ARAMBHA STATE THE YOGI'S MIND BECOMES BRILLIANT, THE BODY BECOMES LUSTROUS AND IT EMITS A DIVINE SMELL.

The majority of practitioners have not even reached this first stage. People will do Sadhana for years and still their body and mouth reeks. This is because they grow up eating meat and it takes years for all the cells to change and for the body to cleanse itself from a cellular level. Also, one has to be emotionally balanced or else emotional upheaval pours toxins into the physical systems. Do not be discouraged. Persevere and you will obtain a lustrous body and a brilliant, discriminative, pure mind. Even if you do not bathe for a few days, the body will still have a sweet odor.

GHATA AVASTHA

72

IN THE SECOND OR GHATA STAGE, THE PRANA AND APANA UNITE AND FLOW THROUGH SUSHUMNA. THE YOGI IS FIXED IN HIS ASANA AND BECOMES WISE AND GOD-LIKE.

73

AT THIS STAGE, WHEN THE VISHNU GRANTHI IS PIERCED, THE YOGI EXPERIENCES THE ANAHATA SOUND OF KETTLE DRUMS RESULTING IN HIGH BLISS.

PARICHAYA AVASTHA

74

IN THE THIRD STAGE, THE PRANA REACHES THE AJNA CHAKRA WHICH IS THE SOURCE OF ALL SIDDHIS AND THE ANAHATA SOUND OF MARKALA IS EXPERIENCED.

75

TRANSCENDING THE HIGHEST SENSUAL AND MENTAL PLEASURE, THE ATMIC BLISS IS EXPERIENCED. IMBALANCE OF THE DOSHAS, PAIN, DISEASE, OLD AGE, HUNGER AND SLEEP ARE OVERCOME.

These Slokas show the progression of the different stages that you undergo. When the Brahma Granthi is pierced, you enter the first stage, which is called the Arambha state. At this point, you experience certain sounds and signs, which are all specific to a certain state of consciousness. Next is the Ghata state, which occurs when the Vishnu Granthi is pierced. At this point, you hear the sound of kettle drums. In the Parichaya Avastha, the third stage, the Prana reaches the Ajna Chakra, which is the source of all Siddhis and the Anahata sound of Markala is experienced. The Markala is a type of instrument. Transcending the highest sensual and mental pleasure, you become free from pain and disease because you have gone beyond base consciousness and body consciousness. You are now identifying with the Higher Reality.

76

WHEN THE RUDRA GRANTHI IS PIERCED, THE PRANA MOVES TO THE SEAT OF ISHWARA. THIS IS THE STAGE OF NISHPATTI AND THE ANAHATA SOUND OF A WELL TUNED VEENA AND FLUTE IS EXPERIENCED.

77

THIS UNION OF INDIVIDUAL AND SUPREME CONSCIOUSNESS IS CALLED RAJA YOGA AND THE YOGI AQUIRES THE POWER OF CREATION AND DISSOLUTION LIKE THAT OF A GOD.

78

THIS RAJA YOGA STATE IS UNINTERRUPTED BLISS BUT MAY NOT NECESSARILY RESULT IN LIBERATION.

79

TO PRACTICE HATHA YOGA AND FALL SHORT OF THE HIGHEST UNION, RAJA YOGA, IS CONSIDERED TO BE A GREAT WASTE.

This Sloka encourages you to persevere until you reach the goal, Self-Realization. It would be a great waste if you barely missed the goal. Hatha Yoga can take you there, to the highest state or Raja Yoga. It is a full, complete system designed to take you to Self-Realization.

80

THE UNMANI STATE IS EASILY REACHED BY FOCUSING THE MIND ON THE AJNA CHAKRA. BY THIS METHOD, EVEN THE UNEDUCATED CAN REACH THE STATE OF RAJA YOGA. THE LAYA PRODUCED THROUGH NADA GIVES IMMEDIATE BLISS.

Here the terms Laya, Raja Yoga and Unmani are synonymous.

81

THE NADA YOGI WHO REACHES SAMADHI THROUGH THE EXPLORATION OF ANAHATA NADA, EXPERIENCES BLISS THAT IS INDESCRIBABLE.

82

THE YOGI SHOULD FOCUS HIS MIND ON THE ANAHATA NADA WHILE CLOSING THE EARS, UNTIL THE MIND REACHES THE STATE OF STILLNESS.

83

THE YOGI BECOMES UNAWARE OF ALL EXTERNAL SOUNDS WITHIN FIF-
TEEN DAYS THROUGH THIS PRACTICE AND EXPERIENCES GREAT HAP-
PINESS.

84

THE ANAHATA NADA THAT IS FOCUSED ON BECOMES LOUDER. EVEN-
TUALLY THE YOGI BECOMES AWARE OF MORE SUBTLE SOUNDS.

85

DIFFERENT ANAHATA SOUNDS ARE HEARD IN DIFFERENT STAGES OF
PRACTICE. IN THE BEGINNING, THE SOUND OF OCEAN IS HEARD,
THEN CLOUDS, KETTLE DRUMS AND JHARJHARA DRUMS. IN THE MID-
DLE STAGE, THE CONCH, GONG AND HORN IS HEARD.

86

IN THE LAST STAGE, THE SOUND OF TINKLING BELLS, FLUTE, VEENA
AND HUMMING OF BEES ARE HEARD AS IF COMING FROM WITHIN THE
BODY.

87

CONTINUE IN THIS MANNER MOVING FROM THE LOUDEST SOUND
LIKE THOSE OF KETTLE DRUMS AND THUNDER TO THE SUBTLER
SOUNDS.

88

EVEN THOUGH THE MIND MAY MOVE FROM THE LOUD TO THE SUB-
TLE AND AGAIN TO THE LOUD, DO NOT LET IT WANDER AWAY TO ANY-
THING ELSE.

89

WHATEVER NADA THE MIND FOCUSES ON, IT BECOMES ABSORBED IN
THAT.

90

JUST AS A BEE IS UNCONCERNED WITH THE FRAGRANCE OF THE
FLOWER WHILE IT IS DRINKING THE HONEY, THE MIND THAT IS
IMMERSED IN NADA LOSES ALL CRAVING FOR SENSUAL ENJOYMENTS.

91

JUST AS AN EXCITED ELEPHANT IS CONTROLLED BY A SHARP GOAD, SO IS THE MIND HABITUATED IN ROAMING IN THE GARDEN OF SENSUAL ENJOYMENTS, CONTROLLED BY ANAHATA NADA.

92

THE MIND THAT IS CAPTIVATED BY ANAHATA NADA ABANDONS ITS RESTLESS NATURE JUST LIKE A BIRD WHOSE WINGS ARE CLIPPED.

93

THE YOGI WHO DESIRES COMPLETE MASTERY OF YOGA SHOULD DEVOTE HIS TOTAL ATTENTION ON THE EXPLORATION OF ANAHATA NADA.

So many analogies are drawn here to express that sensual experiences pale in comparison to the Divine, sublime experience of Anahata Nada.

94

JUST AS A HUNTER CAPTURES A DEER WITH A SNEER AND KILLS IT, SO IS THE MIND CAPTURED AND KILLED BY ANAHATA NADA.

95

THE YOGI SHOULD MEDITATE REGULARLY ON THE NADA BECAUSE IT IS THE BOLT THAT WILL LOCK THE RESTLESS HORSE OF THE MIND.

96

JUST LIKE LIQUID MERCURY IS MADE SOLID WITH SULPHUR, SO IS THE RESTLESS MIND MADE STEADY BY NADA AND ROAMS FREELY IN THE OCEAN OF BRAHMAN.

97

JUST LIKE A SERPENT IS CHARMED BY MUSIC, SO THE MIND CAPTIVATED BY NADA BECOMES STEADY AND UNMOVING.

98

JUST AS FIRE IS EXTINGUISHED WHEN THE WOOD IS BURNT UP, SO THE RESTLESS MIND SUBSIDES IN THE CONCENTRATION ON NADA.

99

JUST AS A DEER, WHEN IT ATTRACTED BY THE SOUND OF BELLS, IS EASILY KILLED BY AN EXPERT ARCHER, SO IS THE MIND BROUGHT UNDER CONTROL BY AN ADEPT NADA YOGI.

100

THE MIND DISSOLVING IN ANAHATA NADA REACHES THE SUPREME STATE OF VISHNU.

101

THE CONCEPT OF SPACE AND DUALITY EXIST AS LONG AS THERE IS AWARENESS OF SOUND. WHEN THIS AWARENESS DISSOLVES AND THE SOUNDLESS STATE IS REACHED, THAT IS THE EXPERIENCE OF BRAH- MAN, THE SUPREME REALITY.

102

WHATEVER IS EXPERIENCED AS ANAHATA NADA IS BUT THE SUBTLE VIBRATION OF SHAKTI. THE ABSOLUTE REALITY IS FORMLESS AND SOUNDLESS.

103

HAVING ATTAINED THE HIGHEST STATE THROUGH THE PRACTICE OF HATHA YOGA, THE YOGI OVERCOMES DEATH AND ABIDES IN THE SUPREME STATE OF RAJA YOGA.

104

MIND IS THE SEED, HATHA IS THE SOIL AND DISPASSION IS THE WATER. BY THESE THREE THE KALPA VRIKSHA, UNMANI AVASTA SPROUTS FORTH.

105

THROUGH THE CONSTANT PRACTICE OF NADA YOGA, ALL KARMAS ARE BURNT UP AND THE PRANA AND CHITTA MERGES IN BRAHMAN.

106

IN THIS UNMANI AVASTHA, THE BODY BECOMES LIKE A LOG AND NOT EVEN THE ANAHATA SOUND OF CONCH OR DRUMS IS HEARD.

107
THAT YOGI, HAVING TRANSCENDED ALL THE STATES OF CONSCIOUS-
NESS AND FREE OF ALL THOUGHTS, IS LIBERATED WITHOUT A DOUBT
AND APPEARS AS IF DEAD.

108
THE YOGI IN SAMADHI TRANSCENDS TIME, IS UNAFFECTED BY KARMA
AND CANNOT BE SUBDUED BY ANYONE.

109
THE YOGI IN SAMADHI, LOSES AWARENESS OF SMELL, TASTE, TOUCH,
SOUND, FORM, HIS BODY AND THAT OF OTHERS.

110
THE YOGI WHO IS NEITHER ASLEEP NOR AWAKE, WHO IS FREE OF
REMEMBERING OR FORGETTING, WHO IS NEITHER ACTIVE NOR INAC-
TIVE, IS INDEED LIBERATED.

Remembering, forgetting, action and inaction are all just modifications of the
mind. They are all effects of the mental fluctuation.

111
THE LIBERATED YOGI IS FREED FROM THE PAIRS OF OPPOSITES OF
HEAT AND COLD, PLEASURE AND PAIN, HONOR AND DISHONOR.

112
THOUGH AWAKE APPEARS TO BE ASLEEP, WHO IS NOT BREATHING YET
REMAINS ALIVE, IS LIBERATED WITHOUT A DOUBT.

113
THE YOGI IN SAMADHI IS INVULNERABLE TO ANY WEAPON, CANNOT
BE HARMED BY ANY BEING AND IS BEYOND THE INFLUENCE OF
MANTRAS OR YANTRAS.

114

AS LONG AS THE PRANA DOES NOT FLOW THROUGH SUSHUMNA, AS LONG AS THE BINDU IS NOT UNDER CONTROL, AS LONG AS THE MIND DOES NOT REFLECT THE PURE LIGHT OF BRAHMAN, THAT PERSON WHO SPEAKS OF SPIRITUAL KNOWLEDGE IS ONLY EXPRESSING HIS DELUSION.

This Sloka cautions that speaking of spiritual knowledge before the mind reflects the pure light of the Soul, is really to perpetuate delusion and magnify one's own ego. That is because such a person will be interpreting the Higher Reality through his own filtered lens. But in essence, what is meant here is to be wary of the person who stands on a pulpit preaching without having first gone through his own awakening.

The most effective teaching is what flows from direct experience. However, even the fully Enlightened Master can only give an indication as to what enlightenment is through his writings and teachings. Each person who is exposed to that teaching receives at his own level of consciousness and fantasy. It is difficult to convey a sensual experience to another person. And it is impossible to convey a transcendental experience. Each person has to experience it for himself. That is why Master Sivananda said that "an ounce of practice is worth more than tons of theory."

Since enlightenment happens in stages, a teacher should teach, with humility but without inhibition, what he has experienced as truth and beneficial to humanity, knowing in his heart that teaching and learning is best for spiritual growth.

Adhidevika: Suffering caused by nature.

Adhyatmika: Suffering caused by oneself.

Adibhautika: Suffering caused by other beings.

Adharas: Receptacle, lower region.

Adinath: Literally means the 'first lord'; primordial Guru; name of Lord Shiva.

Ahata Nada: Sound created by striking two objects.

Ahimsa: One of the Yamas; non-violence, non-injury.

Anahata Nada: The subtle vibrations of Prana experienced by Yogis in a state of meditation.

Ama: Toxins or impurity accumulated in the body.

Amaroli: The drinking of the midstream of urine or applying it on the body as Mudras.

Annamaya Kosha: The food sheath.

Anuloma Viloma: Alternate nostril breathing.

Apana: Downward or outward movement of Prana

Arambha: First stage of hearing the internal sound or Anahata Nada.

Asana: A steady and comfortable pose.

Avatar: Descent or incarnation of Supreme Consciousness as God. e.g. Rama, Krishna.

Bandhas: Practices that create a psychomuscular energy lock which redirects the flow of energy or Prana in the body and locks it into a specific area.

Bhadrasana: "Gracious pose;" a sitting posture.

Bhajan: Songs that are sometimes philosophical or in praise of God, rendered in a spirit of devotion.

Bhakti Yoga: The Yoga of devotion and love for God.

Bhasti: The cleansing of the colon. One of the Kriyas in Hatha Yoga.

Bhastrika: The bellows breath in which inhalation and exhalation is forcibly and in equal proportions, like the pumping of the bellows.

Bhramari: Breathing practice in which a humming sound is produced during exhalation like that of the black bee.

Bindu: Point or seed of potential energy and consciousness; nucleus.

Brahma: The creator.

Brahmacharya: Celibacy; disciplining of the senses; living in awareness of Brahman.

Brahmachari: Celibate; one who lives a life of purity and directs his energy to study.

Brahman: Pure consciousness; the One without a second.

Chakra: Pranic or psychic centers in the subtle body.

Chitta: Mind-stuff; subconscious mind.

Dana: Charity; giving.

Dhanurasana: Bow pose.

Dharma: Righteous way of living; one of the Purusharthas or treasures of life.

Dhatus: The different tissues of the physical body; altogether there are seven Dhatus.

Dhauti: Cleansing of the stomach.

Deva: Divine being; higher force or power.

Ghata: Second stage of hearing the Anahata Nada.

Gomukhasana: Cow's face posture.

Gorakshasana: A variation of Bhadrasana.

Grihastha: Householder, the second stage of life.

Gunas: Quality of nature; threefold capacity of manifest Shakti, Prakriti or nature. These are Tamas, Rajas and Sattwa.

Guptasana: Another name for Siddhasana.

Hatha Yoga: A step-by-step science of Yoga that takes you from the very basic, starting with proper health and culminating with Self Realization.

Jalandhara Bandha: Throat lock that prevents Prana from flowing out.

Jala Neti: One of the Shatkarmas; nasal cleansing with water.

Japa: Continuous repetition of your Mantra.

Jnana Yoga: Yoga of self enquiry.

Ida: Major Nadi running on the left side of the spine.

Ishta Devata: Personal deity, chosen ideal of the Supreme.

Kaala: Time: death; Yama.

Kalaa: That which radiates.

Kalpa: One day of Brahma.

Kapalabhati: One of the six cleansing exercises in Hatha Yoga called the cleansing breath. Emphasis is on exhalation just like when you are blowing your nose in rapid succession.

Kapha: one of the three humours or Doshas according to Ayurveda; phlegm, mucus.

Karma: Action; law of cause and effect. Cleansing exercises.

Karma Yoga: Yoga of selfless action.

Khechari: What moves in the sky.

Kevala Kumbhaka: Spontaneous suspension of the breath.

Kirtan: Singing the name and glory of God.

Klesha: Afflictions or pain.

Kriya: Cleansing action; Yogic practice.

Kukkutasana: Cockerel pose.

Kumbhaka: Breath retention.

Kundalini: The primordial cosmic energy that lies dormant at the base of the spine.

Kurmasana: The tortoise pose.

Lakshmi: Goddess of wealth; consort of Vishnu.

Laya: Dissolution; merging; absorption of mind.

Madhyama: Mental vibration.

Manas Prakriti: The constitution of the mind, i.e Sattva, Rajas and Tamas.

Manipura Chakra: Literally means "city of jewels;" one of the seven psychic and pranic centers, located in the region of the navel.

Manomaya Kosha: The mental sheath located in the astral body.

Manonmani: Literally means "mind without mind;" state of Samadhi.

Mantra: The vibrational representation of a specific manifestation of God.

Matsyendrasana: The spinal twist pose.

Mayurasana: The peacock pose.

Mudra: Literally means "gesture;" physical, mental and psychic attitude which expresses and channels cosmic energy within the mind and body.

Muktasana: Another name for Siddhasana.

Mula Bandha: The contraction of the perineum. Drawing the energy up and preventing the Apana from flowing down.

Murccha: Fainting; one of the main Kumbakhas in Hatha Yoga.

Nada Yoga: Science of sound vibration, that leads to the goal of Self Realization.

Nadam: Sound vibration.

Nauli: Abdominal massage; One of the Shatkarmas in which the rectus abdomini muscles are contracted and isolated vertically.

Neti: Nasal cleansing with either water or a waxed string; one of the Shatkarmas.

Nishpatti: The fourth stage of hearing the Anahata sound.

Niyamas: Observances that help to maintain the vows of Yamas.

Ojas Shakti: Vitality; sublimated sexual energy.

Padmasana: Lotus pose.

Para: Supreme. The highest undifferentiated state of vibration.

Paschimottanasana: "Back stretching pose;" Forward bending posture.

Pashyanti: The second stage of differentiation of Nada Brahman as this universe.

Pingala: One of the main Nadis culminating in the right nostril that is heating as it channels the solar energy.

Pitta: One of the three Doshas or humours; bile.

Plavini: Gulping breath in which air is swallowed into the stomach; one of the main Kumbakhas in Hatha Yoga.

Prakriti: Nature; manifested Shakti; vehicle of Purusha.

Prana: Vital life-force sustaining and permeating the whole of creation.

Pranamaya Kosha: The energy sheath; one of the five sheaths of the individual.

Pranayama: The ability to control and direct Prana; technique of breathing and breath retention.

Puja: Worship; rituals expressing one's devotion and adoration to God.

Purusha: The Supreme being; another term for God.

Raga: Attachment that is binding; attraction.

Rama: Incarnation of the preserving aspect of God known as Vishnu.

Raja Yoga: The Yoga of the study and control of the mind through concentration and meditation; the eightfold path known as Ashtanga Yoga as formulated by Maharishi Patanjali.

Rajas: One of the qualities of nature and mind expressed as dynamism; movement or agitation.

Rudra Granthi: Psychic knot located in Ajna Chakra.

Sadhana: Conscious self-effort to improve and elevate one's consciousness.

Sahajoli: Practice of Vajroli by a woman.

Samadhi: The eighth stage of Ashtanga Yoga where the Yogi transcends the limitations of body, mind and intellect and wakes up in the fourth state of consciousness and experience the Self as Divine.

Samana: The Prana that functions in the middle region of the body to digest food.

Sampoorna Yoga: The Yoga of fullness; The intelligent integration of the different aspects of Yoga to accelerate one's evolution in a balanced and harmonious way.

Samskara: Impressions formed from thoughts and actions that manifest as personality traits, life after life.

Sanyasin: Renunciate; one who lives a life of detachment for the purpose of Self-Realization.

Saraswati: Goddess of learning and arts; consort of Brahma.

Satchitananda: Absolute existence, knowledge and bliss.

GLOSSARY

Satsanga: Association with the wise seeking self knowledge.

Sattwa: One of the three Gunas expressed as purity, light, knowledge, etc.

Savasana: Corpse pose.

Shakti: Cosmic energy; creative, potential force.

Shaktipat: Transmission of Shakti from Guru to disciple.

Shambhavi Mudra: Concentration of mind while gazing at the mid-eyebrow center.

Shastras: Authoritative treatises on any subject, especially pertaining to science or religion.

Shatkriyas: The six Hatha Yoga techniques of cleansing: Neti, Dhauti, Nauli, Bhasti, Trataka, Kapalabhati.

Shiva: Pure consciousness; Lord of the Yogis.

Shukra Dhatu: Reproductive cells.

Siddha: An adept; a master.

Siddhasana: Pose of perfection.

Simhasana: The Lion pose.

Sitkari: One of the main Kumbakhas in Hatha Yoga.

Sloka: A verse of praise.

Sushumna: Main Nadi that runs along the center of the spine.

Sutra Neti: Nasal cleansing with thread; one of the Shatkarmas of Hatha Yoga.

Sutras: Thread; aphorism; the least number of words that convey an idea or truth.

Swastikasana: Auspicious pose; meditative posture similar to Siddhasana.

Suryabheda: Vitality stimulating the breath; one of the main Kumbhakas in Hatha Yoga.

Tala: Rhythmic cycles.

Tamas: One of the three Gunas that is characterized by laziness, dullness; everything that is gross and dense.

Tantra Yoga: The Yoga that deals with the Divine Shakti.

Tapas: Sadhana or self-effort to discipline the senses and purify the mind.

Tejas: Fire or luster, brilliance.

Trataka: One of the Shatkarmas; technique of gazing steadfastly upon an object such as a candle flame, Mandala or Yantra.

Tridoshas: The three bodily constitutions referred to in Ayurveda as Vata, Pitta and Kapha.

Udana: Pranic air current in the area of the throat and face.

Uddiyana Bandha: Abdominal retraction lock; drawing in of the abdomen upwards and towards the spine after exhaling.

Ujjayi: Psychic breath performed by contracting the epiglottis producing a light sonorous sound.

Unmani: literally means "no mind" or "without mind;" state of Samadhi; consciousness devoid of finite mind.

Unmani Avastha: mindless state of a Yogi.

Uttanakurmasana: Stretching tortoise pose.

Vajrasana: Thunderbolt pose.

Vajroli Mudra: "Thunderbolt attitude." In this Mudra the muscles of the male sexual organ and lower urinary tract are contracted to redirect sexual energy upwards. A practice of Hatha Yoga.

Vedas: Eternal laws that flow through the minds of purified beings called

Rishis which explain and regulate every aspect of life from supreme reality to worldly affairs.

Vanaprastha: One who leads the third stage of life.

Vasana: A deep-rooted desire in the unconscious mind.

Vasistha: One of the seven eternal beings or Sapta Rishis; author of many Vedic hymns; family Guru of king Raghu Dinasty. His teachings are recorded in the Yoga Vasistha, one of the greatest expositions of Jnana Yoga.

Vata: One of the three Doshas; with air and ether as its constituting elements.

Vijnanamaya Kosha: The intellectual sheath.

Vaikhari: The fourth or grossest level of manifestation of vibration that can be perceived by the senses.

Viparita Karani: One of the Mudras in Hatha Yoga where the body is upside down.

Virasana: The hero's pose.

Vishuddi Chakra: Psychic center located at the throat.

Vishnu: One of the holy trinity known as the cosmic preserver.

Vishnu Granthi: Psychic "knot" in Anahata Chakra.

Vishnu Mudra: In this Mudra, the index and middle fingers of the right hand are bent towards the palm. This Mudra is used to do Anuloma Viloma Pranayama.

Veena: A classical Indian instrument.

Vritti: Mental modification.

Vyana: Diffusive or outward moving air.

Yajna: Fire ceremony in which oblations and Mantras are offered into a sacrificial fire.

Yamas: Self-restraints; first limb of Raja Yoga.

Yantra: A precisely calculated geometrical symbol representing a specific aspect of Shakti.

Yogi: An adept practitioner of Yoga, who has reached the goal of Self Realization.

Yogini: A female adept practitioner of Yoga, who has reached the goal of Self Realization.

Yoni Mudra: Also known as Shanmukhi Mudra; symbolically closing of the seven gates of perception in the head with the fingers of both hands. A specific hand gesture symbolizing the Divine Mother. It is also used during meditation.

SRI YOGI HARI

Sri Yogi Hari *is a Master of Hatha, Raja and Nada Yoga. He is well-known and respected around the world as a competent and inspiring teacher. Sri Yogi Hari comes from the Sivananda lineage. When he met his Gurus, Swami Vishnu-Devananda and music master Swami Nada-Brahmananda in 1975, he retired from worldly life and spent seven years in the Sivananda Ashram where he immersed himself fully in Yoga Sadhana.*

Sampoorna Yoga is the fruit of Sri Yogi Hari's tireless striving for perfection in his practice and teaching. This is the Yoga of fullness through an intelligent integration of Hatha, Raja, Karma, Bhakti, Jnana and Nada Yoga to purify and harmonize all aspects of the human personality so that the light of the soul shines forth in all its Divine splendor. His approach is deep, simple and practical, and helps people from every background to live a richer, happier life based on lasting Yogic values. The basic teaching is that health, peace and joy are already within you. Sampoorna Yoga can help you to realize this and lift the veils so that you abide in your true nature.

Sri Yogi Hari has produced 32 audio tapes and 30 CDs of chanting, Bhajans, Kirtan, Mantras and Shlokas. He has also compiled a book with the transliteration and meaning of the songs on all the tapes and CDs. Yogi Hari's Bhajans, Kirtans and Mantra chanting instill peace and joy in the hearts of listeners. The soul stirring philosophies of the songs, sung in melodious Ragas and Talas, calm the mind and lift one to a heightened state of bliss.

He has also produced a series of "Nada Yoga at Home" on video and DVD. Audio Visual technology has made it possible to transmit this ancient mystical knowledge as if the Guru is actually in your presence. The Hatha Yoga videos and DVD productions are given the same care in orchestration as the musical tapes. The result is an experience of health, relaxation and peace of mind, body and spirit.

Regular classes, seminars, Sadhana week, teachers training courses and Satsang are given by Yogi Hari at his Ashram in Miramar, Florida. His inspirational teachings, in all their different aspects, lead to the ultimate goal of living the Divine Life right here and now through a healthy body, healthy mind and high aspirations.

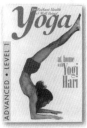

YOGA DVDs, VIDEOS AND AUDIO SERIES

You can now have private classes in your home with an adept Yoga Master guiding you each step of the way. Whether you are a complete beginner or you are already practicing Yoga, these DVDs, videos and audios will help you progress quickly. Each tape is a complete class starting with an invocation, continuing with breathing, warming up and strengthening exercises. This is followed by Yoga postures that are taught in a systematic manner that work on the entire body to tone and strengthen all the systems. The class culminates in a guided deep relaxation. Each cassette has calming background music.

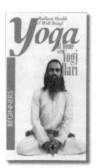

BEGGINERS. 60 MINS

This Beginners DVD & video is a complete session of a well blended yoga formula to yield all the benefits of health and well being. Breathing and warming up exercises and beautifully orchestrated Yoga postures give a complete and balanced workout.

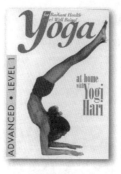

INTERMEDIATE LEVEL 2
90 MINS

An adventure with your body and mind. You will be doing more pranayama and asanas and experiencing a smooth flow from one asana to another. Through regular practice, you will enjoy radiant health and well being, and you will better able to cope with daily stress.

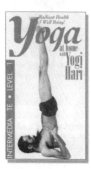

INTERMEDIATE LEVEL 1
90 MINS

Greater emphasis is place in breathing, with the introduction of Kapalabathi (cleansing breath and Anuloma Viloma (alternate nostril breath). The Headstand is introduced as well as variations on basis postures.

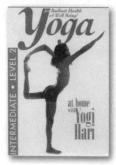

ADVANCED LEVEL 1
120 MINS

Deeper understanding of the limitless science of Hatha Yoga for perfect health and well being. Great emphasis on pranayama. Experiencing the prana will take you to a new level of inner awarness. This video challenges you to keep progressing.

"If you are looking for the essence of a Hatha Yoga practice on tape, look no further." - YOGA INTERNATIONAL.

TO ORDER CALL: 1-800-964-2553

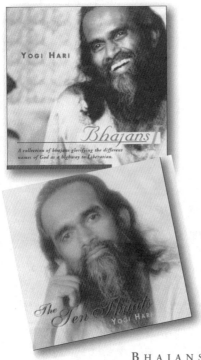

Bhajans, *Kirtans and* Chants

🕉

Yogi Hari has produced 32 audio tapes and 30 CDs of chanting, bhajans, kirtan, mantras and slokas. He has also compiled a book with the transliteration and meaning of the songs on all the tapes and CDs.

Yogi Hari's bhajans, kirtans and mantra chanting instill peace and joy in the hearts of listeners. The soul stirring philosophies of the songs, sung in melodious Ragas and Talas, calm the mind and lift one to a heightened state of bliss.

BHAJANS

These bhajans are poems written by Enlightened beings and set to music and sung with devotion by Yogi Hari. They are either devotional in nature, glorifying God in all aspects, or philosophical, reminding us that life is the most valuable treasure and that every moment should be utilized to attain Self-Realization or Liberation. The Saints had a special ability to condense and summarize a complex and abstract philosophy into a few explicit verses. When rendered by a Yogi, a Saint or a spiritual aspirant, they have the capacity to heal the body and to lift the mind out of depression, leaving one with a feeling of peace and joyfulness. This is why is important to intgrate the listening and chanting of bhajans into one's practice.

SATSANG AND CHANTING

Singing the names of the Lord, or Kirtan, is considered the easiest way to God realization. The mind becomes easily controlled. The heart melts with love and devotion. Transformation of character takes place. The devotee becomes a channel for the expression of the divine. Wherever he is, there is peace & joy.

TO ORDER CALL: 1-800-964-2553

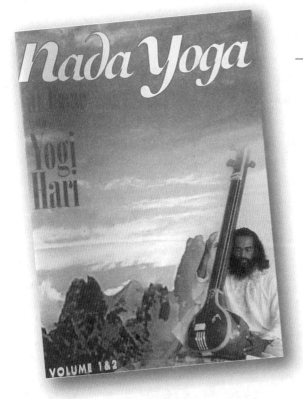

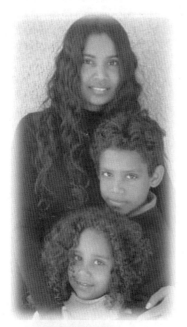

Meditations by
CHITTRA

CHITRA SUKHU a mother of two and the daughter of Yogi Hari and Leela Mata has practiced meditation since the age of four, and is an accomplished Indian Classical dancer in the ancient style of Bharata Natyam. She started her company New Age Kids, Inc. with the desire to help create a generation of healthy, well balanced individuals with a sense of self.

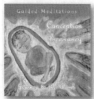

Guided Meditation for Conception and Pregnancy

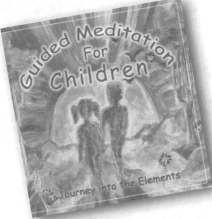

Guided Meditation for Children

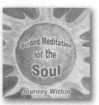

Guided Meditation for the Soul

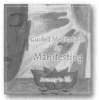

Giuded Meditations for Manifesting

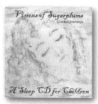

Visions of Sugarplums-Guided Journeys

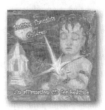

Positive Thoughts for Children

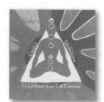

To Unleash Your Full Potential. Chakras: the key to the mysteries of life.